MRI Atlas of MS Lesions

M. A. Sahraian, E.-W. Radue

MRI Atlas of MS Lesions

With the collaboration of A. Gass, S. Haller, L. Kappos,
J. Kesselring, J.-I. Kira, K. Weier

Springer

Prof. Dr. med. Mohammad Ali Sahraian
Assistant Professor of Neurology
Department of Neurology
Tehran University of Medical Sciences
Hassan Abad Square
Sina Hospital
Tehran-Iran
msahrai@sina.tums.ac.ir

Prof. Dr. med. Ernst-Wilhelm Radue
Head of Department of Neuroradiology
University Hospital Basel
Petersgraben 4
4031 Basel
Switzerland
eradue@uhbs.ch

Additional material to this book can be downloaded from http://extras.springer.com

ISBN 978-3-642-44781-5 Springer Berlin Heidelberg New York

Springer is a part of Springer Science + Business Media
springer.com

Softcover re-print of the Hardcover 1st edition 2008

Editors: Dr. Ute Heilmann/Annette Hinze, Heidelberg, Germany
Desk editor: Meike Stoeck, Heidelberg, Germany
Cover design: Frido Steinen-Broo, eStudio Calamar, Spain
Production & Typesetting: LE-TEX Jelonek, Schmidt & Vöckler GbR, Leipzig, Germany
Printed on acid-free paper 21/3180/YL – 5 4 3 2 1 0

To our wives Barbara and Niloofar
and our children Pascal, Geraldine and Amir hossien

Preface

Magnetic resonance imaging (MRI) has greatly increased our understanding about multiple sclerosis (MS) during the last two decades, and is now considered to be the imaging of choice for diagnosis and in vivo monitoring of the disease.

New diagnostic criteria allow us to demonstrate dissemination of MS pathology in space and time by MRI, thus making early diagnosis and treatment possible. Exclusion of other possible pathologies is a main step in MS diagnosis. Also in this context, MRI plays an important role. Despite its high sensitivity, MRI is not a specific tool for diagnosing MS, and almost any alteration in cerebral white matter may change the signal intensity on T2-weighted images. Nevertheless, understanding MS lesion characteristics, patterns on different sequences, and topography of lesions in the central nervous system help to determine if MS is the best diagnosis for a patient who has presented with signs and symptoms of white matter involvement.

The present book aims at demonstrating MS lesions in different sequences of conventional MRI, and shows examples of typical and atypical lesions. The main idea for collecting the images in this atlas is to show the diversity of MS lesions in different sequences of conventional MRI. There is a summarized introduction at the beginning of each chapter, followed by selected images in different sequences demonstrating MS lesions in different shapes, sizes, and locations. A teaching point has been added to the images as a "Note" in order to increase the information resulting from them. Revised McDonald criteria and some of the most important differential diagnoses have been discussed in two separate chapters. The images have been selected out of thousands of MRI images, and we hope that this *MRI Atlas of MS Lesions*, which is accompanied by a learning CD, provides valuable tools for clinicians and radiologists who are interested in MS for a better depiction of lesions, avoiding pitfalls, and demonstrating dissemination in space and time by MRI.

Acknowledgement

We would like to thank Alexandra Palatini for her secretarial work on the book and her organization skills during the project. Without her assistance, this book would not have been possible.

We also wish to thank Pascal Kuster, Stefan Traud, Alain Thoeni, and Verena Koch for their support in selecting and preparing the images.

M.A. Sahraian
E.-W. Radue

Contents

Contributors

Prof. Dr. med. Achim Gass
Department of Neurology-Neuroradiology
University Hospital Basel
Petersgraben 4
4031 Basel
Switzerland

Dr. med. Sabine Haller
Department of Neuroradiology
University Hospital Basel
Petersgraben 4
4031 Basel
Switzerland

Prof. Dr. med. Ludwig Kappos
Head of Outpatient Clinic Neurology-Neurosurgery
University Hospital Basel
Petersgraben 4
4031 Basel
Switzerland

Prof. Dr. med. Jürg Kesselring
Head of Department of Neurology
and Neurorehabilitation Center
7317 Valens
Switzerland

Prof. Dr. med. Jun-Ichi Kira
Head of Department of Neurology
Neurological Institute
Graduate School of Medical Sciences
Kyushu University
Japan

Prof. Dr. med. Ernst-Wilhelm Radue
Head of Department of Neuroradiology
University Hospital Basel
Petersgraben 4
4031 Basel
Switzerland

Prof. Dr. med. Mohammad Ali Sahraian
Assistant Professor of Neurology
Department of Neurology
Tehran University of Medical Sciences
Hassan Abad Square
Sina Hospital
Tehran-Iran

Dr. med. Katrin Weier
Department of Neurology-Neuroradiology
University Hospital Basel
Petersgraben 4
4031 Basel
Switzerland

How to Read the Atlas

In order to receive maximum information from this book, we highly advise you to have a look on the introductory part of each chapter. There you will find some basic information on each topic, followed by images sorted to show the lesions in different shapes, sizes, and locations, starting from the posterior fossa and continuing to supratentorial structures.

It should be noted that our intent was not to elaborate on all the details on each image. There may be several findings, but we have tried to demonstrate the most important ones according to the topic.

Each image is described in a legend giving additional explanations to the reader as well as important clinical information (correlation lesions/clinical presentation, lesions/course of the disease) under "note".

You will find the basic principles about correct detection of multiple sclerosis (MS) lesions in different sequences, so as to avoid pitfalls.

This atlas is accompanied by a complementary CD on which you will find selected images of different patients with MS. You will have the possibility to select MS lesions out of several suggested areas. Your selection, the correct answer, as well as training remarks, will be shown subsequently.

1 MS Lesions in T2-Weighted Images

M.A. Sahraian, E.-W. Radue

1.1 Introduction

Multiple hyperintense lesions on T2- and PD-weighted sequences are the characteristic magnetic resonance imaging (MRI) appearance of multiple sclerosis (MS). The majority of the lesions are small, although they can occasionally measure several centimeters in diameter. Focal MS lesions are usually round or oval in shape and relatively well circumscribed.

MS lesions may occur in any part of the central nervous system where myelin exists, but lesions around the ventricles and the corpus callosum are highly suggestive. Other common sites of involvement are subcortical and infratentorial regions (Ge 2006). Although MS is a white matter disease, a subset of lesions may involve gray matter including the cerebral cortex, thalamus, and basal ganglia (Ormerod et al. 1987). Cortical involvement has been described in several pathological studies (Brownwell et al. 1962; Peterson et al. 2001), but these lesions may be missed on conventional MRI due to similarities in signal intensities of MS lesions and gray matter or partial volume effect of cerebrospinal fluid within the adjacent sulci (Kidd et al. 1999).

Postmortem studies have demonstrated a close correlation between the lesions seen on pathological examinations and the lesions seen on T2-weighted MRI (Stewart et al. 1984; De Groot et al. 2001). T2 hyperintensities are not specific, and almost any alteration in the brain tissue composition can change signal intensity. Inflammation, demyelination, gliosis, edema, and axonal loss will increase the signal intensity, without any specific pattern (Bruck et al. 1997).

Most of the lesions – especially in the early stages of the disease – are discrete on conventional MRI, although diffuse changes throughout the normal-appearing white matter (NAWM) have been demonstrated by nonconventional MR techniques such as magnetization transfer imaging (MTI) (Ostuni et al. 1999), diffusion-weighted imaging (DWI) (Ciccarelli et al. 2002), and MR spectroscopy (De Stefano et al. 2002). Conventional T2-weighted MR images may also demonstrate diffuse, large, and irregular hyperintensities with poorly defined borders around the ventricles, especially adjacent to the occipital horn. They are known as dirty-appearing white matter (DAWM) and have been reported in 17% of the patients with remitting-relapsing multiple sclerosis (RRMS) (Zhao et al. 2000).

Acute T2 lesions may show a halo of less striking hyperintensity, probably consistent with edema that resolves over time, and they reach their final size within about 6 months.

With ongoing disease, new lesions or enlargement of preexisting lesions can be seen to occur simultaneously with the shrinkage of previously acute plaques. Most T2 lesions develop without clinical symptoms, but most clinical relapses are associated with new lesions on MRI (Smith et al. 1993; Thorpe et al. 1996). On average, MS patients will develop four or five new MRI lesions per year, with great variability among individuals (Paty 1988).

Both cross-sectional and short-term longitudinal correlations between T2 lesion load and clinical impairment are generally poor (Rovaris et al. 2003; Barkhof 1999). Lack of pathological specificity for the extent of tissue destruction, inability of conventional MRI to detect damage in NAWM, limitations of the expanded disability status scale (EDSS), and occurrence of lesions in clinically "silent" areas are some of possible explanations for such a clinicoradiological paradox (Goodin 2006).

T2 lesions have a specific value in predicting the outcome of the patients presenting with clinically isolated syndrome (CIS). CIS patients with normal cerebral MRI at presentation have only an 11% risk of another clinical attack in the next 10 years, whereas those with two or more cerebral lesions have a considerably higher risk (90%) (O'Riordan et al. 1998). Changes in the number and volume of T2 lesions have been used as surrogate markers in clinical trials of new therapeutic agents. These measures are based on the evaluations of serially obtained images and generally require image acquisition according to a standardized protocol (Simon et al. 2006).

This chapter deals with typical as well as atypical MS lesions on T2-weighted images, presenting MS lesions in different patterns, sizes, and locations.

1.2 Shape and Size

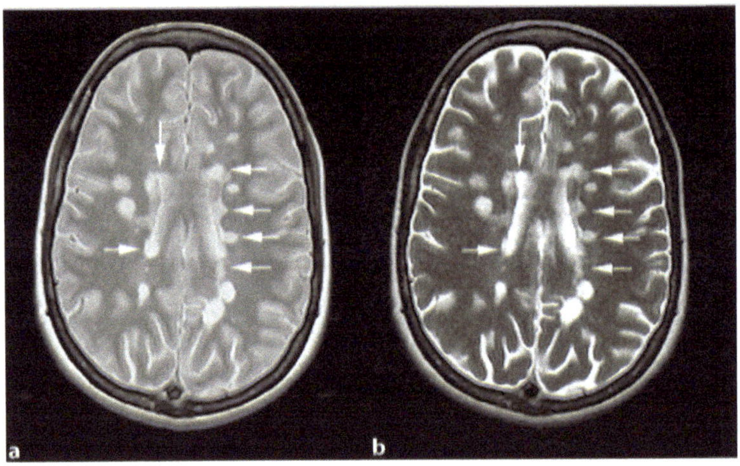

Fig. 1.1 Axial proton density (PD)- (**a**) and T2-weighted (**b**) images of a patient with remitting-relapsing multiple sclerosis (RRMS) demonstrate classic MR appearance of the disease. Note: Multiple hyperintense lesions (plaques) with periventricular predominance are the classic MRI feature of MS (*arrows*)

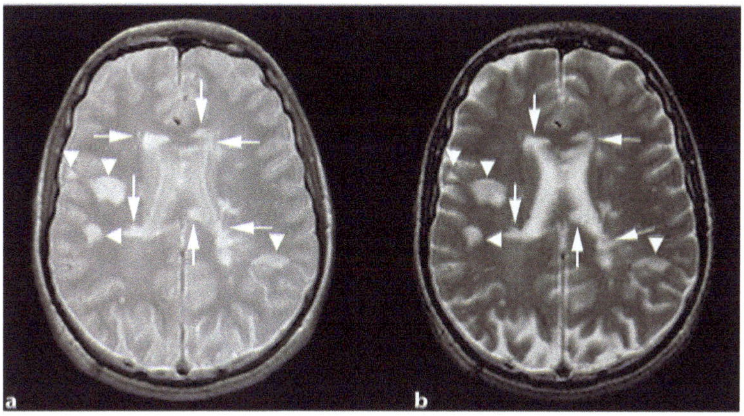

Fig. 1.2 Axial PD- (a) and T2-weighted (b) images demonstrate MS plaques in different areas of the cerebral hemisphere. Note: MS lesions can occur in different locations of the central nervous system. The most common locations are periventricular (*arrows*), juxtacortical (*arrowheads*), corpus callosum, and infratentorial structures

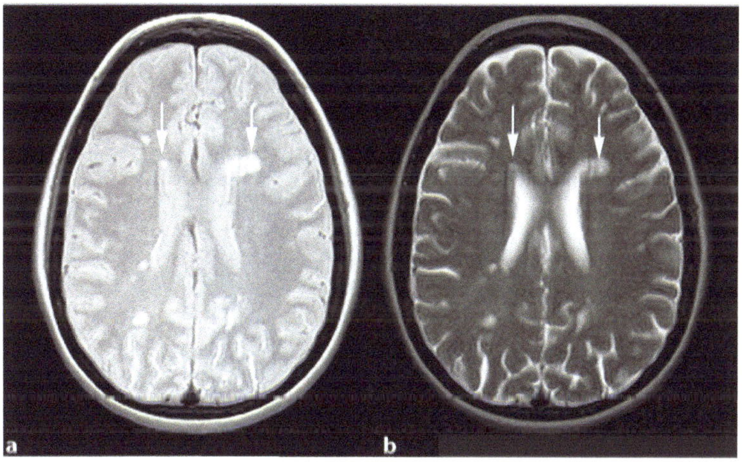

Fig. 1.3 Axial PD- (a) and T2-weighted (b) images demonstrate typical periventricular lesions in MS (*arrows*). Note: Periventricular lesions are defined as the lesions that are attached to the walls of the ventricles

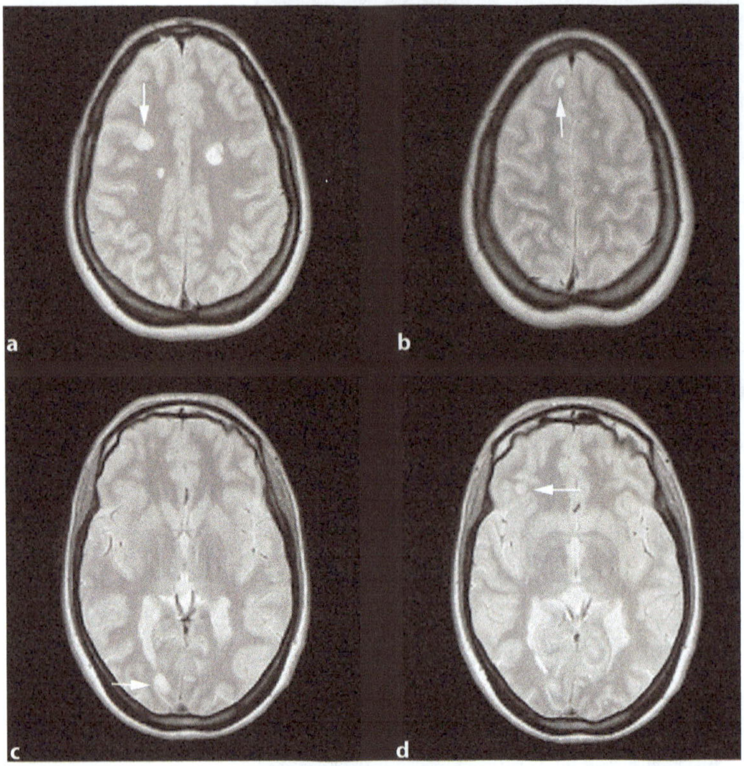

Fig. 1.4 Axial PD- (**a**) and T2-weighted (**b**) images demonstrating juxtacortical lesions in parietal (**a**), frontal (**b, d**) and occipital lobes (**c**) (*arrows*). Note: Juxtacortical lesions are defined as the lesions that touch the cerebral cortex

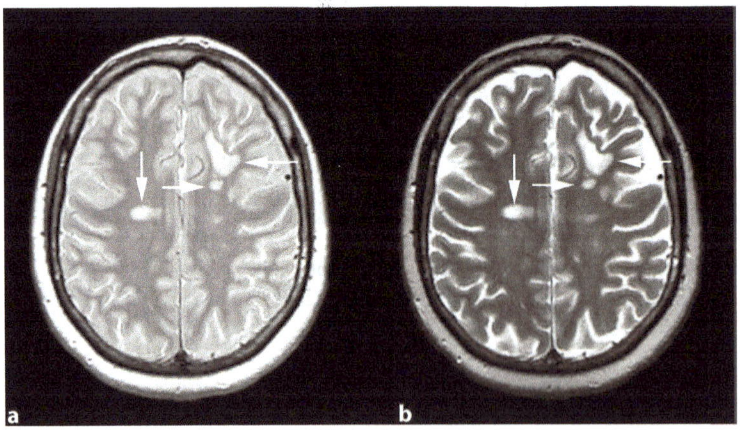

Fig. 1.5 Axial PD- (**a**) and T2-weighted (**b**) images of a patient with RRMS, demonstrating different shapes of the lesions (*arrows*). Note: MS lesions are usually oval or round in shape, but other complex and irregular patterns may also be seen in this disease. In fact, there is no characteristic pattern on T2-weighted images that is specific for MS

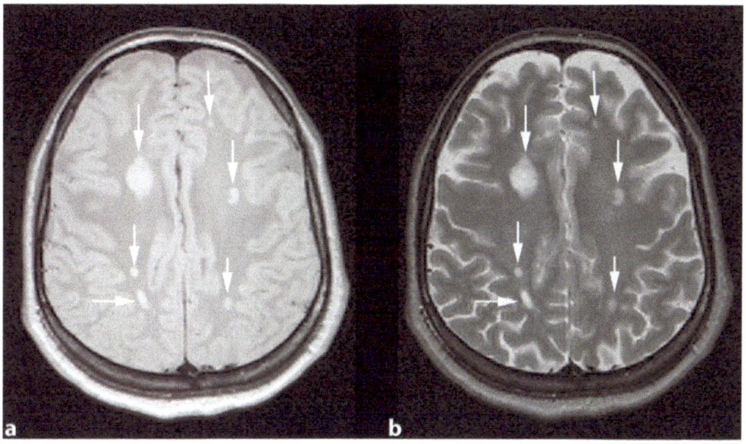

Fig. 1.6 Axial PD- (**a**) and T2-weighted (**b**) images of a patient with MS demonstrate lesions of different sizes (*arrows*). Note: MS lesions are usually small, but the diameter may vary from a few millimeters to several centimeters

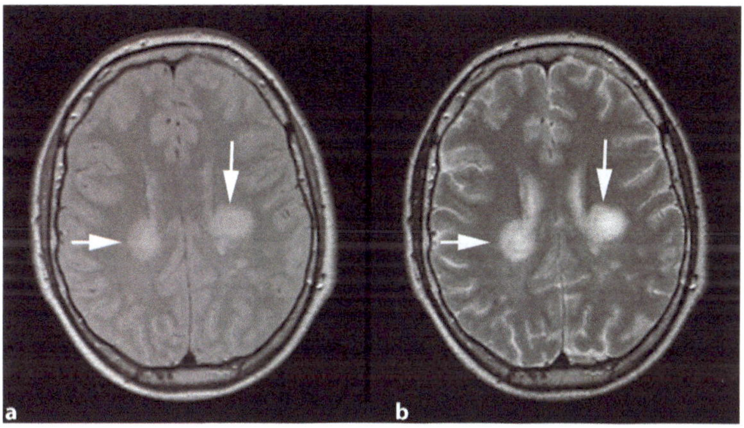

Fig. 1.7 Axial PD- (**a**) and T2-weighted (**b**) images of a patient with RRMS demonstrate lesions of different sizes. Two of the lesions are bilateral, periventricular, and relatively large (*arrows*). Note: The average lesion size has been reported to be 7 mm in nominal diameter, and most MS lesions are smaller than 1 cm in diameter

1.3 Location

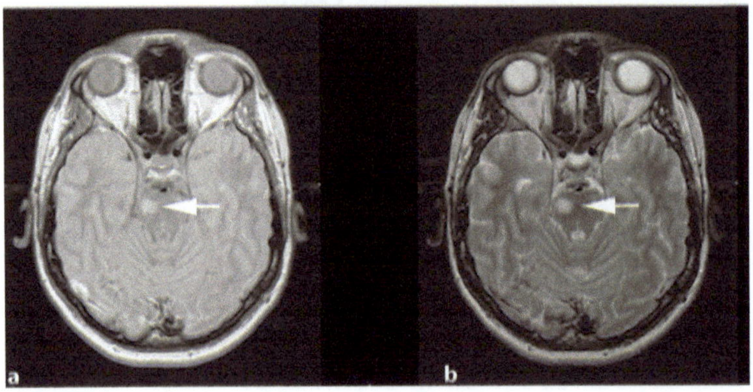

Fig. 1.8 Axial PD- (**a**) and T2-weighted (**b**) images demonstrate a lesion in the upper part of the pons (*arrows*). Note: Infratentorial lesions may be seen in any part of these structures, but lesions are most commonly seen in the pons, cerebellum, and cerebellar peduncles

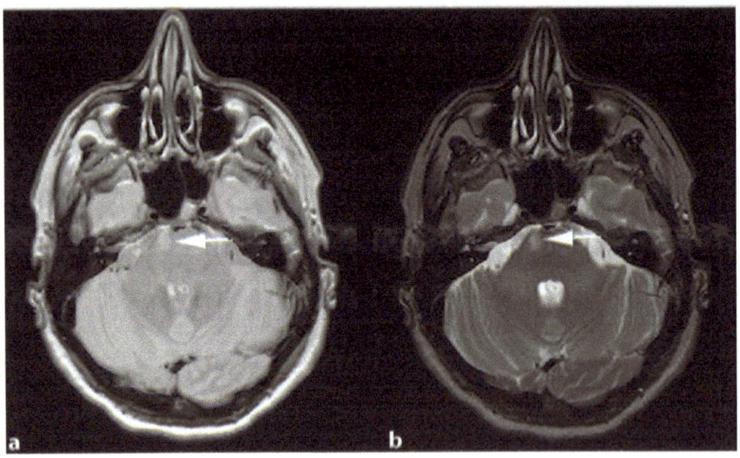

Fig. 1.9 Axial PD- (**a**) and T2-weighted (**b**) images show a lesion in the surface of the pons (*arrows*). Note: Some brainstem lesions may be superficial abutting the subarachnoid space. In contrast to this, abnormalities in the center of the pons are more characteristic in small vessel disease

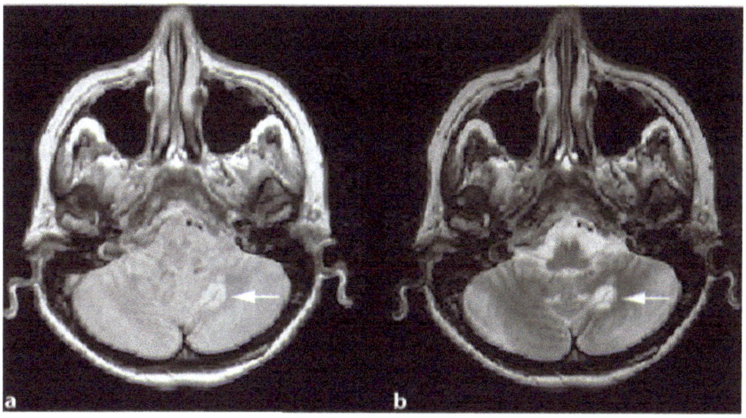

Fig. 1.10 Axial PD- (a) and T2-weighted (b) images of a patient with MS demonstrate a cerebellar lesion (*arrows*). Note: Lesions may occur in any part of the cerebellar white matter. About 50% of MS patients may have one or more lesions in this area

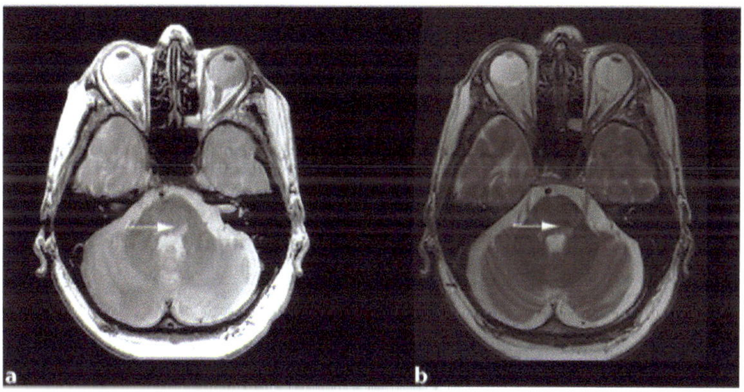

Fig. 1.11 Axial PD- (a) and T2-weighted (b) images demonstrate a lesion in the floor of the 4th ventricle (*arrows*)

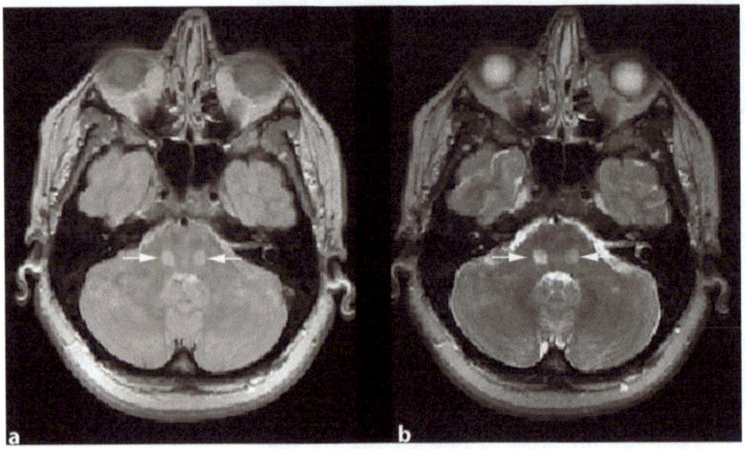

Fig. 1.12 Axial PD- (a) and T2-weighted (b) images demonstrate two bilateral, relatively symmetrical lesions in the pons (*arrows*). Note: Symmetric lesions are not usually seen in MS. The lesions are bilateral rather than symmetrical, but in rare cases symmetrical lesions may be seen in the cerebral hemispheres, brainstem, or cerebellar peduncles

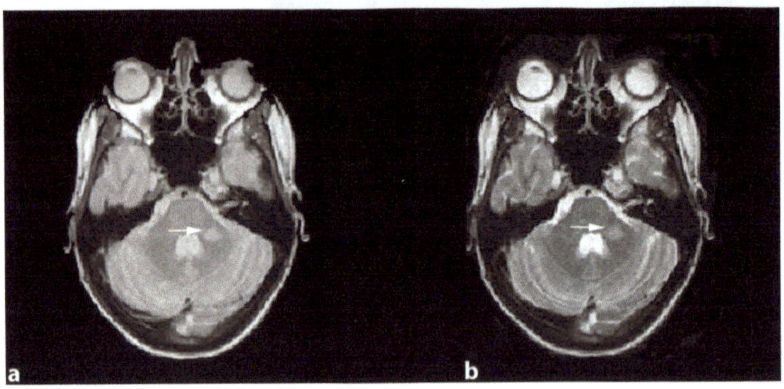

Fig. 1.13 Axial PD- (a) and T2-weighted (b) images of a patient with MS demonstrate a large lesion involving pons and middle cerebellar peduncle (*arrows*). Note: In MS and some other inflammatory diseases the middle cerebellar peduncles are preferentially affected. The reason is not clear

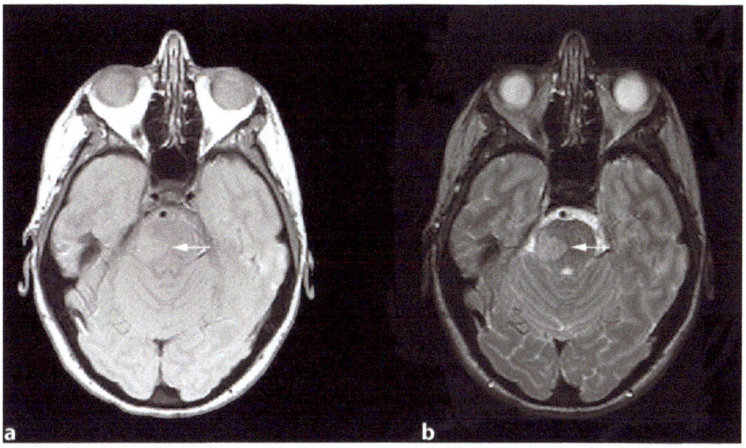

Fig. 1.14 Axial PD- (**a**) and T2-weighted (**b**) images of a patient with RRMS demonstrate a relatively large lesion in the posteroalateral part of the pons (*arrows*)

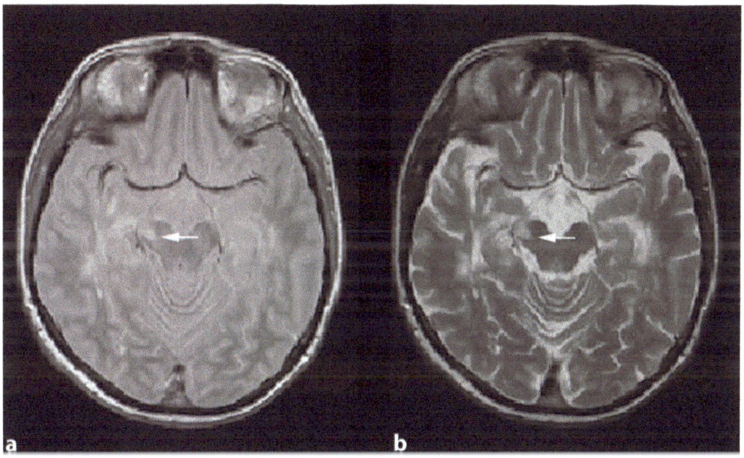

Fig. 1.15 Axial PD- (**a**) and T2-weighted (**b**) images of a patient with RRMS demonstrate a lesion in the cerebral peduncle. The border of the lesion towards the cerebral spinal fluid (CSF) is not clearly defined (*arrows*)

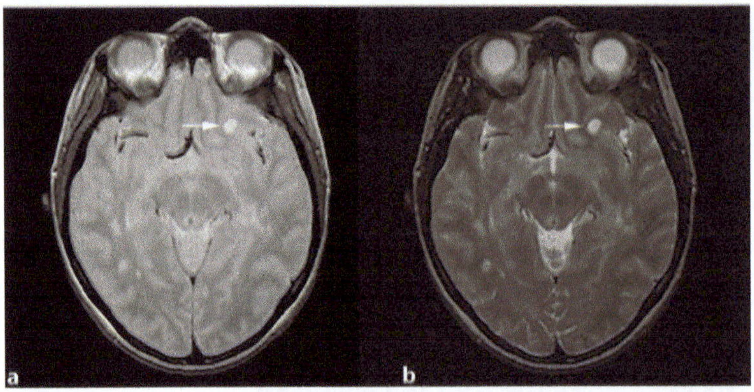

Fig. 1.16 Axial PD- (**a**) and T2-weighted (**b**) images demonstrate a lesion in the base of left frontal lobe (*arrows*)

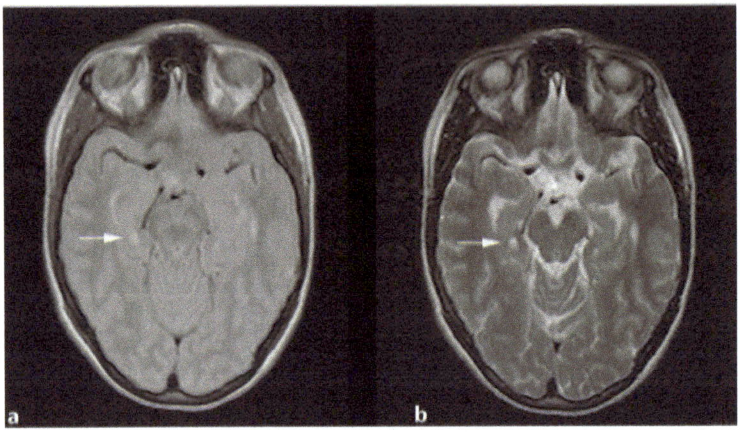

Fig. 1.17 Axial PD- (**a**) and T2-weighted (**b**) images of a patient with MS demonstrate a lesion in the juxtacortical area of the temporal lobe (*arrows*)

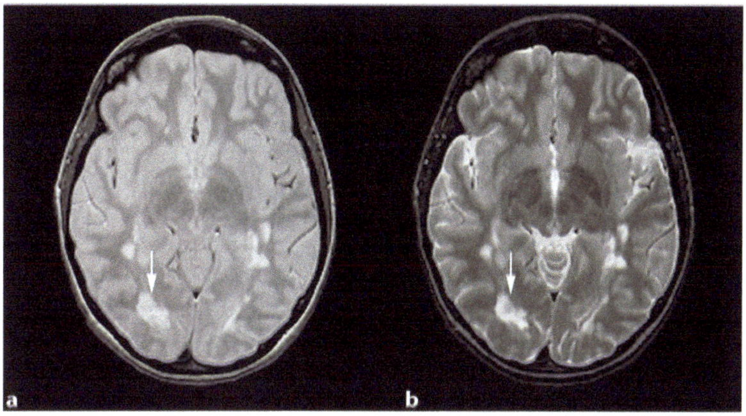

Fig. 1.18 Axial PD- (**a**) and T2-weighted (**b**) images of a patient with MS demonstrate a relatively large lesion in the right occipital lobe (*arrows*)

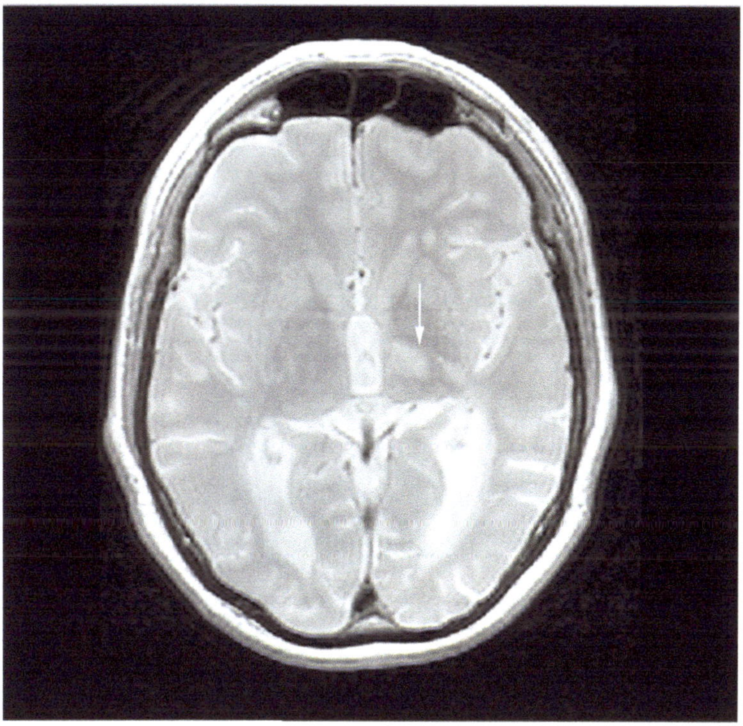

Fig. 1.19 Axial PD-image of a patient with RRMS, demonstrating a thalamic lesion (*arrow*). Note: MS lesions may be seen in thalamus and other gray matter structures (cerebral cortex and basal ganglia). The presence of lesions in such areas does not rule out MS

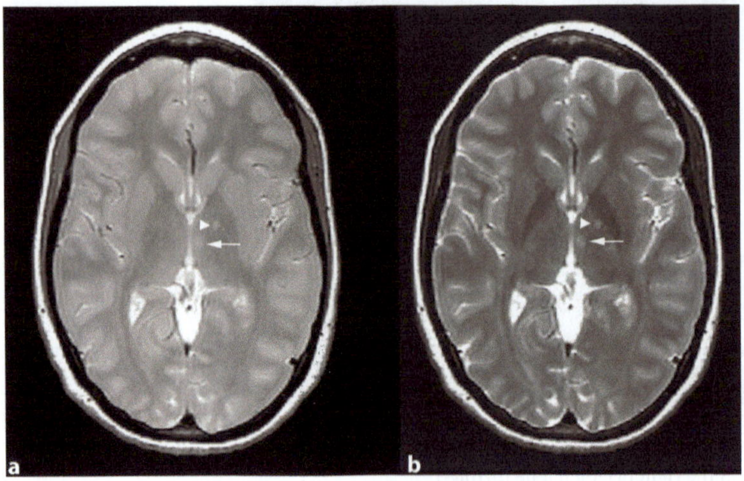

Fig. 1.20 Axial PD- (a) and T2-weighted (b) images of a patient with MS demonstrate a thalamic lesion attached to the third ventricle (*arrows*). This localization is quite rare in MS. Another lesion attached to the internal capsule has been demonstrated by the *arrowhead*

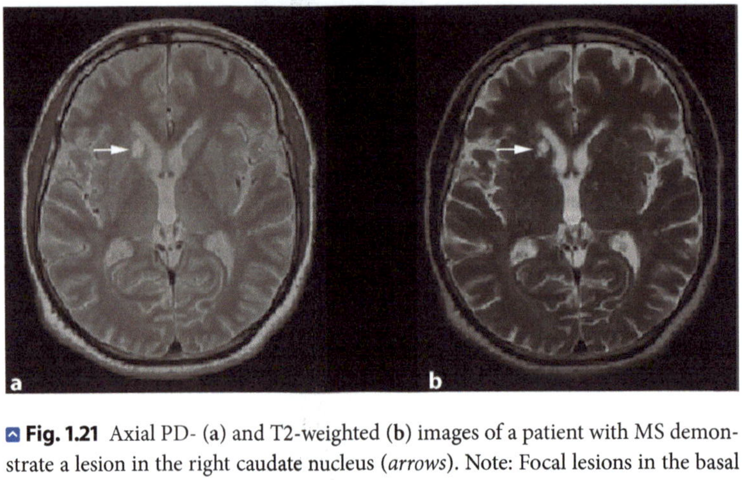

Fig. 1.21 Axial PD- (a) and T2-weighted (b) images of a patient with MS demonstrate a lesion in the right caudate nucleus (*arrows*). Note: Focal lesions in the basal ganglia are not usually seen in MS, although the presence of such a lesion does not exclude the diagnosis

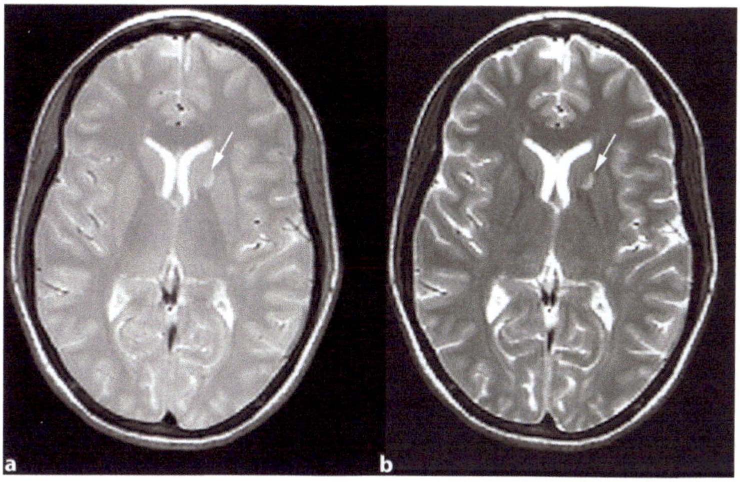

Fig. 1.22 Axial PD- (**a**) and T2-weighted (**b**) images of a patient with MS demonstrate a lesion in the left internal capsule (*arrows*). Note: Lesions of the internal capsule are sometimes seen in MS. Since vascular lesions may frequently involve this region, they are of little diagnostic value in differentiating these two pathologies

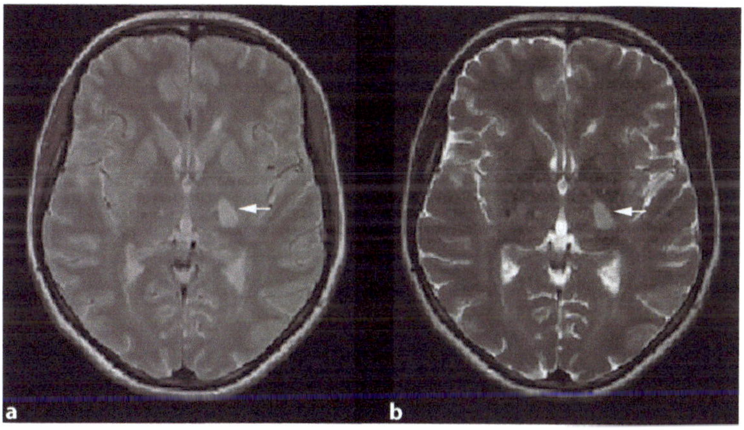

Fig. 1.23 Axial PD- (**a**) and T2-weighted (**b**) images of a patient with MS demonstrate a large lesion in the posterior limb of the left internal capsule (*arrows*)

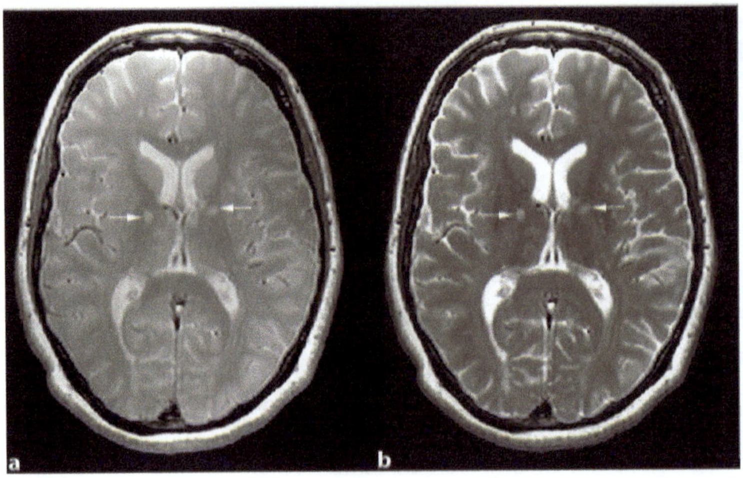

Fig. 1.24 Axial PD- (**a**) and T2-weighted (**b**) images of a patient with RRMS demonstrate bilateral, nonsymmetrical lesions in the genu of both internal capsules (*arrows*)

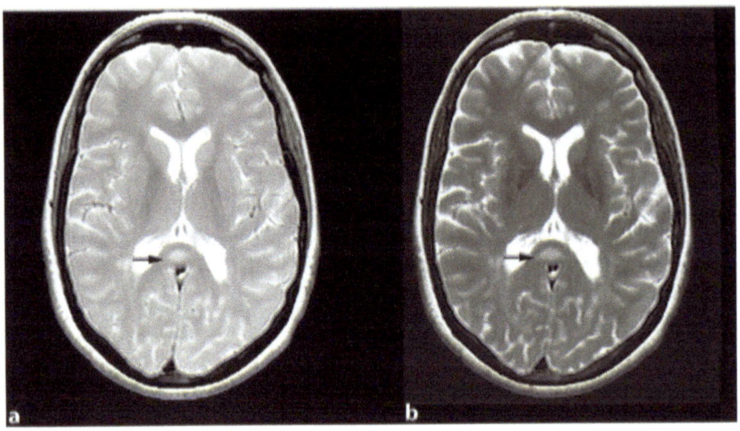

Fig. 1.25 Axial PD- (**a**) and T2-weighted (**b**) images of a patient with RRMS demonstrate a lesion in the splenium of the corpus callosum (*arrows*). Note: Lesions within the corpus callosum are commonly seen in MS but are rarely associated with vascular causes of white matter diseases. This can help in differentiating MS from other pathologies

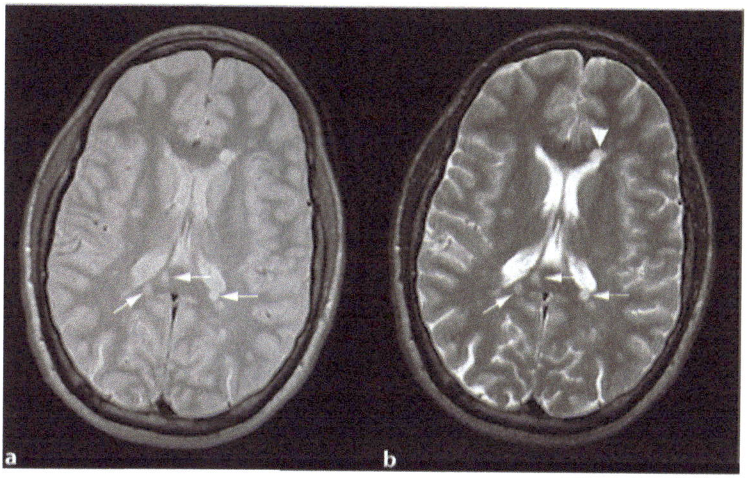

Fig. 1.26 Axial PD- (**a**) and T2-weighted (**b**) images of a patient with RRMS demonstrate several lesions in the genu (*arrowhead*) and splenium of the corpus callosum (*arrows*)

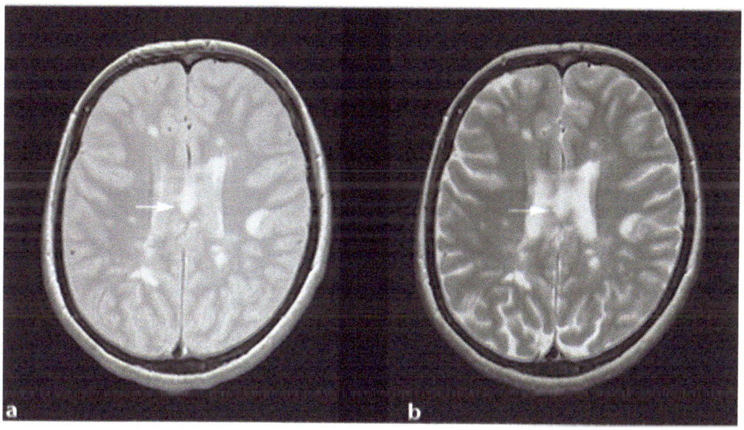

Fig. 1.27 Axial PD- (**a**) and T2-weighted (**b**) images of a patient with MS show several lesions in both cerebral hemispheres. A large lesion is demonstrated in the body of the corpus callosum (*arrows*)

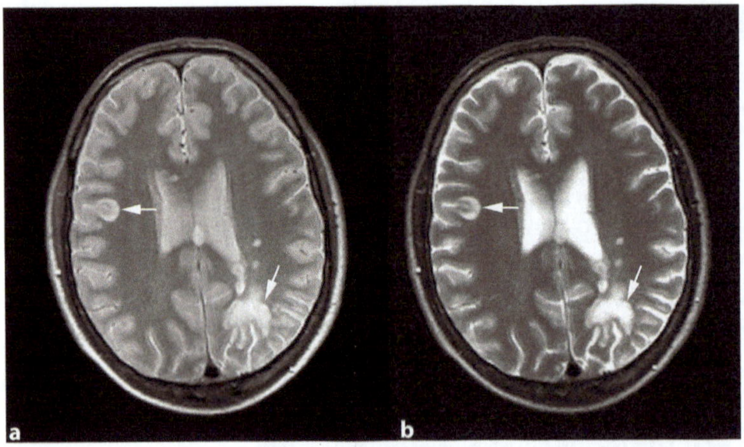

Fig. 1.28 Axial PD- (a) and T2-weighted (b) images of a patient with RRMS show involvement of subcortical U fibers (*arrows*). Note: MS lesions tend to involve U fibers in the juxtacortical area. In Binswanger's disease U fibers are usually spared

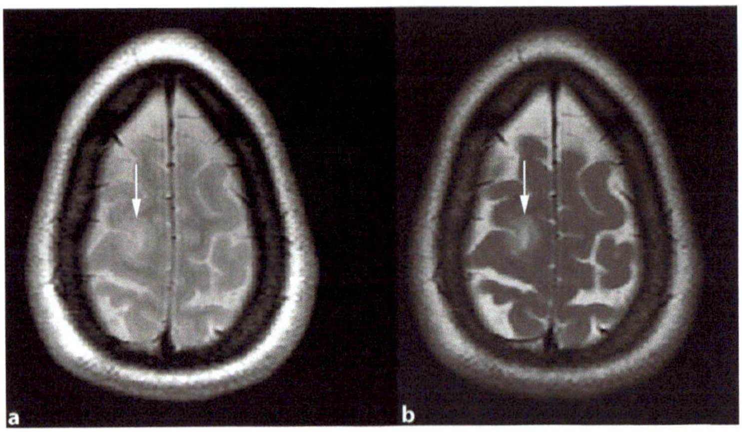

Fig. 1.29 Axial PD- (a) and T2-weighted (b) images of a patient with RRMS demonstrate a lesion in the vertex of the right cerebral hemisphere (*arrows*)

1.4 Follow-Up

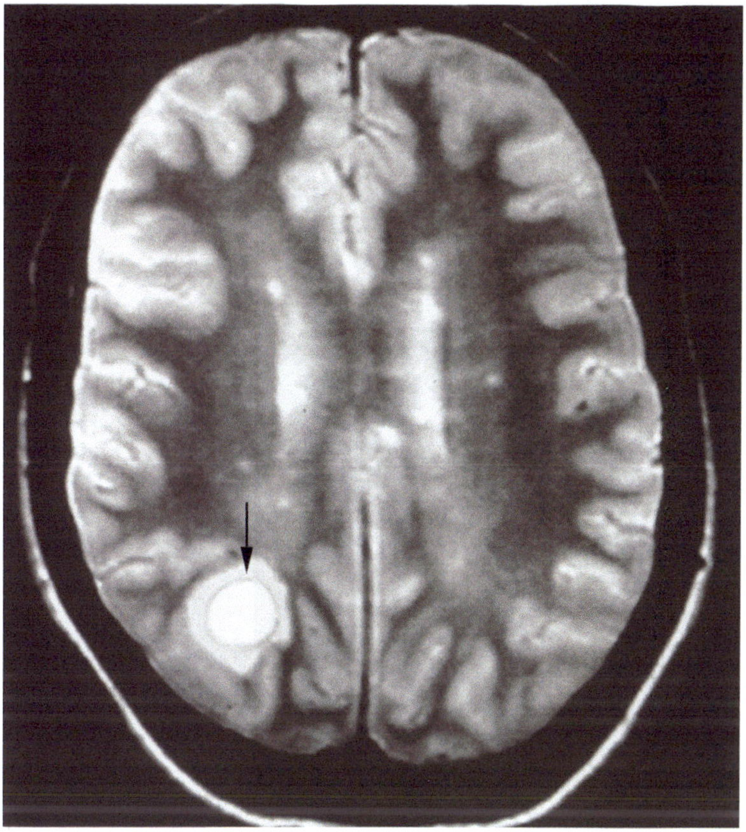

Fig. 1.30 Axial T2-weighted image of a patient with RRMS, demonstrating an acute lesion in the occipital area. Note: Acute lesions may have a complex pattern in T2-weighted images with a central hyperintensity, surrounded by an iso- to hypointense ring (*black arrow*) and another hyperintense signal around the isointense ring

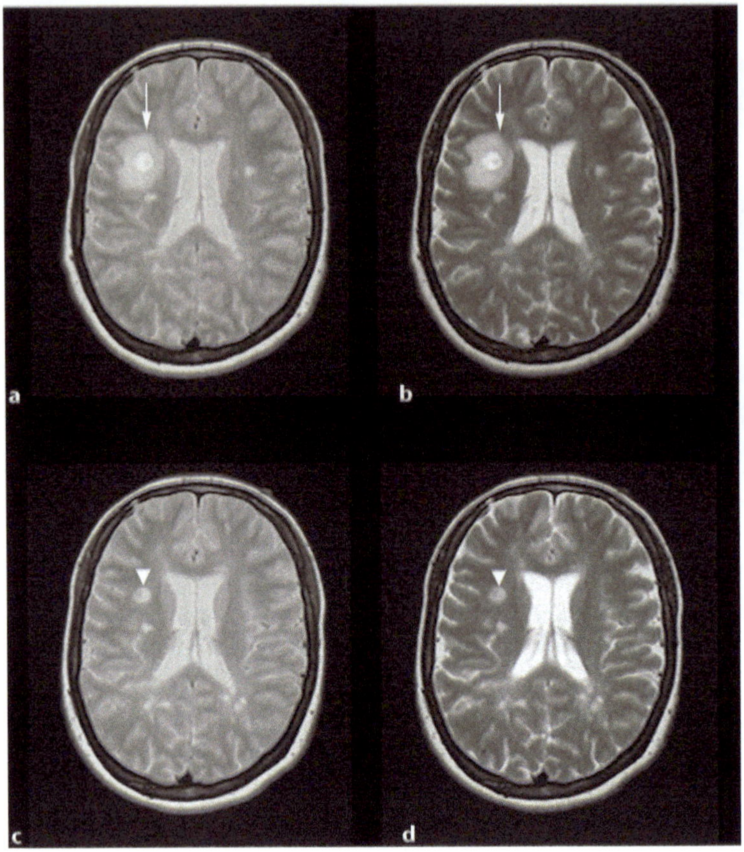

Fig. 1.31 Axial PD- (**a**) and T2-weighted (**b**) images of a patient with MS and their follow-up images (**c,d**) demonstrate an acute lesion (*arrows*) reduced in size, with resolution of edema after 6 months (*arrowheads*). Note: New T2 lesions usually contract and their intensity reduces as edema resolves and some tissue repair occurs

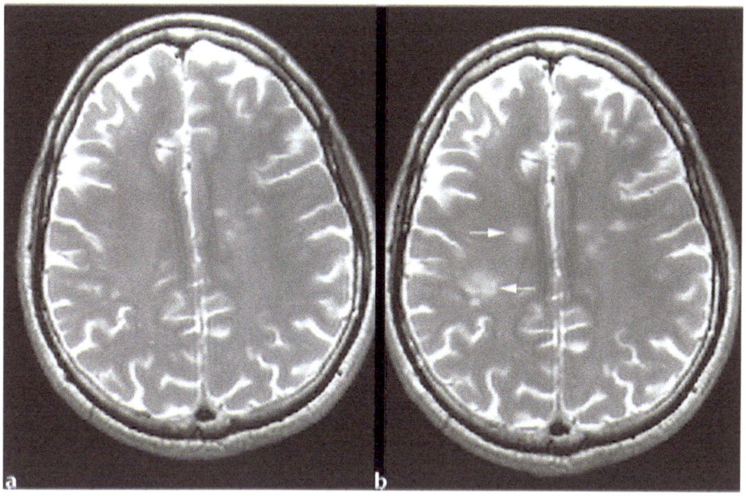

Fig. 1.32 Axial T2-weighted image of a patient with RRMS at baseline (**a**) and a follow-up image after 1 year (**b**) demonstrate two new lesions (*arrows*). Note: New T2 lesions represent new inflammatory activity and are a surrogate marker in clinical trials

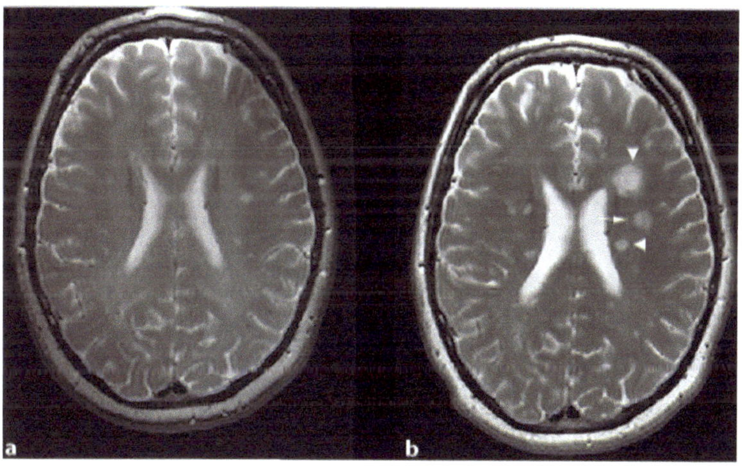

Fig. 1.33 Axial T2-weighted image of a patient with RRMS at baseline (**a**) and a follow-up image after 1 year (**b**) demonstrate several new lesions (*arrowheads*). One of the lesions has been enlarged compared to the baseline (*arrow*). Note: Previously noted lesions may enlarge (i.e., enlargement by about 20% in lesional area in a single slice). Enlarging lesions are due to new inflammatory activity, and in clinical trials on MS they are usually also considered as new lesions

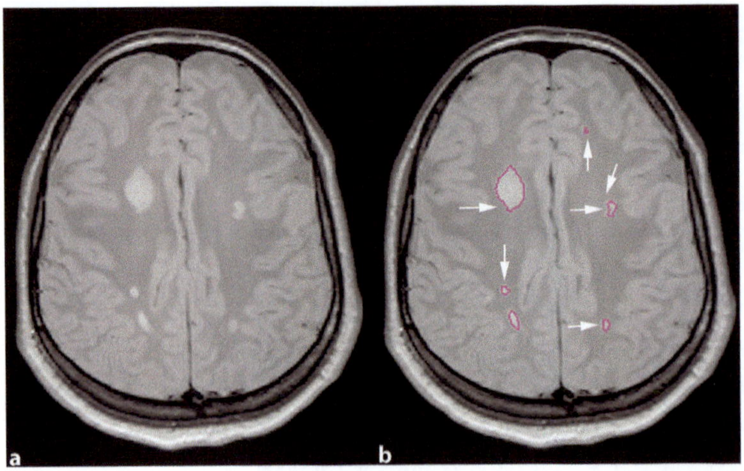

Fig. 1.34 Axial PD- (a, b) images of a patient with MS demonstrate semiautomated segmentation of lesions in order to measure T2 lesion load (*arrows*). Note: The extent of lesions seen on T2-weighted images is commonly referred to as T2 burden of disease and is used as a surrogate outcome marker in clinical trials on MS

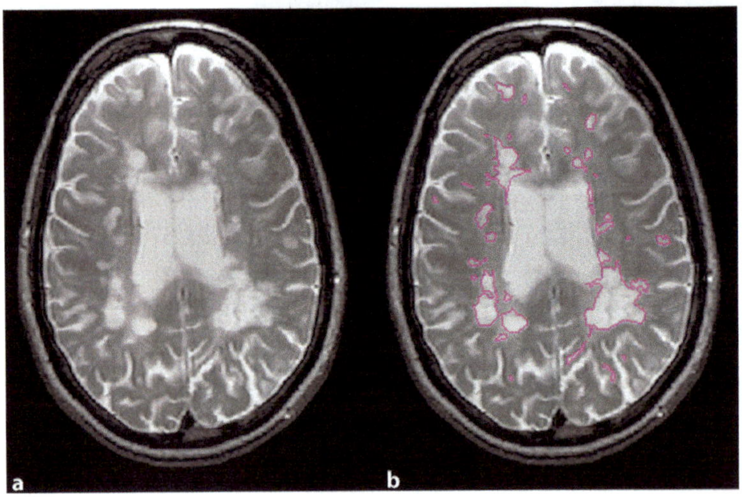

Fig. 1.35 Axial T2-weighted image (a) of a patient with RRMS demonstrates some small and large lesions. The segmentation of the lesions has been shown in **b**. This patient has a high lesion volume load. Note: T2 lesion volume load may be mild (few lesions), moderate (multiple lesions, partially confluent), and severe (many, confluent lesions)

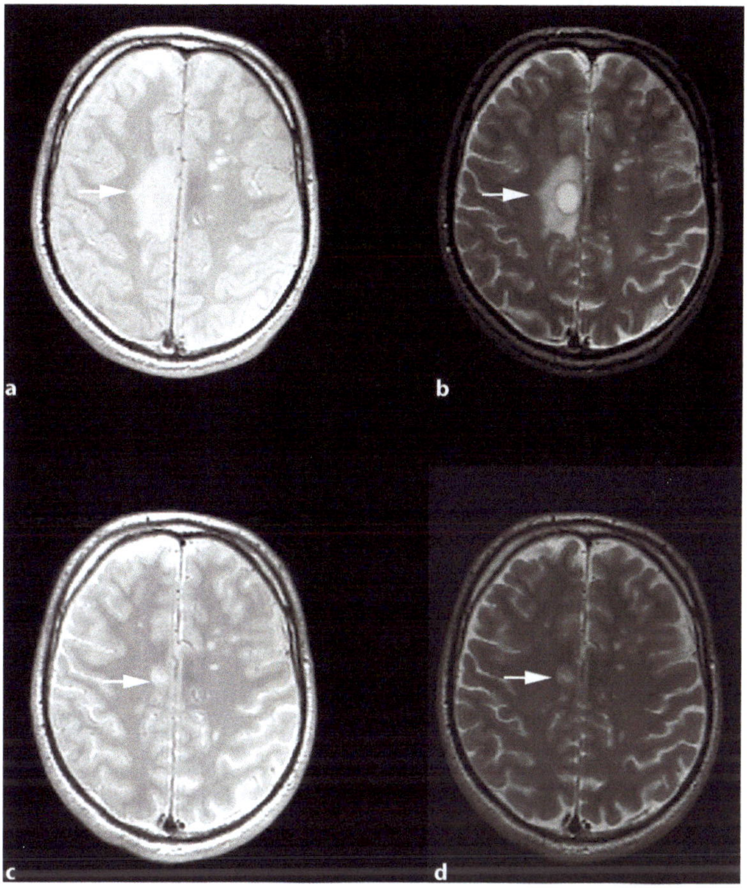

Fig 1.36 Axial PD- (**a**) and T2-weighted (**b**) images of a patient with RRMS demonstrate a large acute lesion involving cortex and subcortical area (*arrows*). Follow-up images (**c**,**d**) after 1 year demonstrate that the lesion has significantly resolved but is still present (*arrows*)

1.5 Normal Appearing White Matter

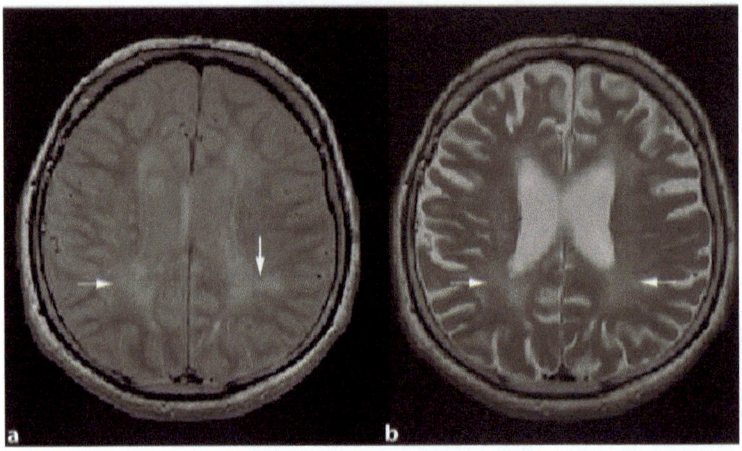

Fig.1.37 Axial PD- (**a**) and T2-weighted (**b**) images of a patient with RRMS demonstrate dirty-appearing white matter (*arrows*). Note: In contrast to normal-appearing white matter (NAWM), subtle, abnormal, and diffuse signal intensity changes are often seen on T2-weighted images, which have been referred to as dirty-appearing white matter. Their signal intensity is slightly higher than NAWM but lower than real lesions

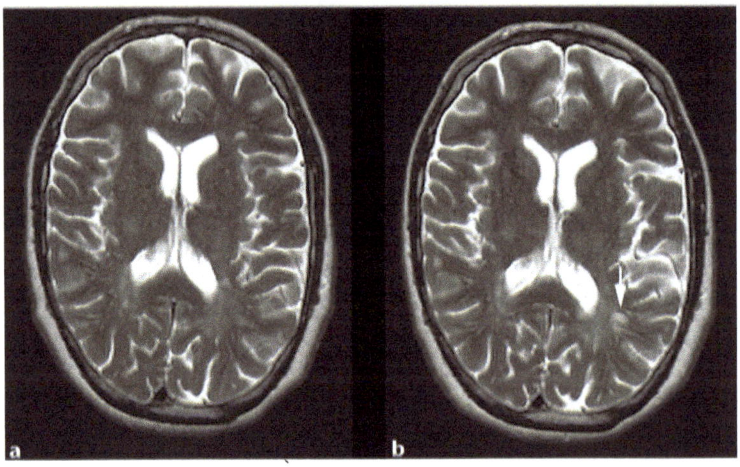

Fig. 1.38 Axial T2-weighted image of a patient with RRMS (**a**) demonstrates dirty-appearing white matter. The follow-up image after 1 year (**b**) demonstrates a new lesion that has been formed in this area (*arrow*)

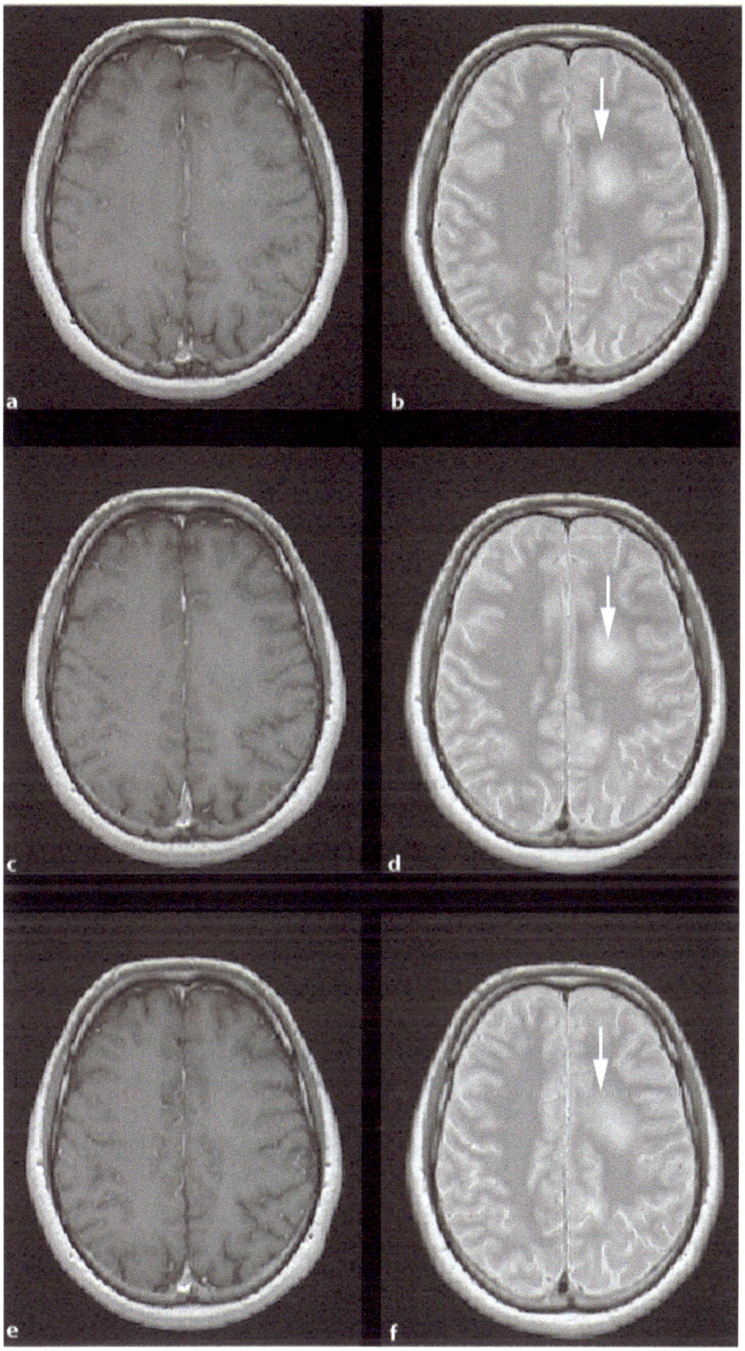

Fig. 1.39 Axial T1-weighted (**a**,**c**,**e**) and PD (**b**,**d**,**f**) images of a patient with RRMS demonstrate a relatively large and nonhomogeneous lesion on three consecutive slices (*arrows*). The lesion is nonenhancing and does not have sharp borders. Note: MS lesions – especially chronic ones – have sharp borders. Some lesions may have fuzzy borders, mostly in their acute state

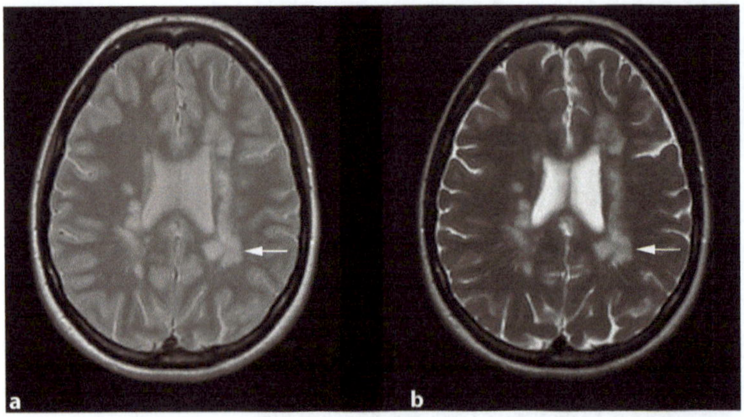

Fig. 1.40 Axial PD- (a) and T2-weighted (b) images of a patient with MS demonstrate confluence of lesions (*arrows*). Note: In MS, several small lesions may fuse to form a large, confluent lesion

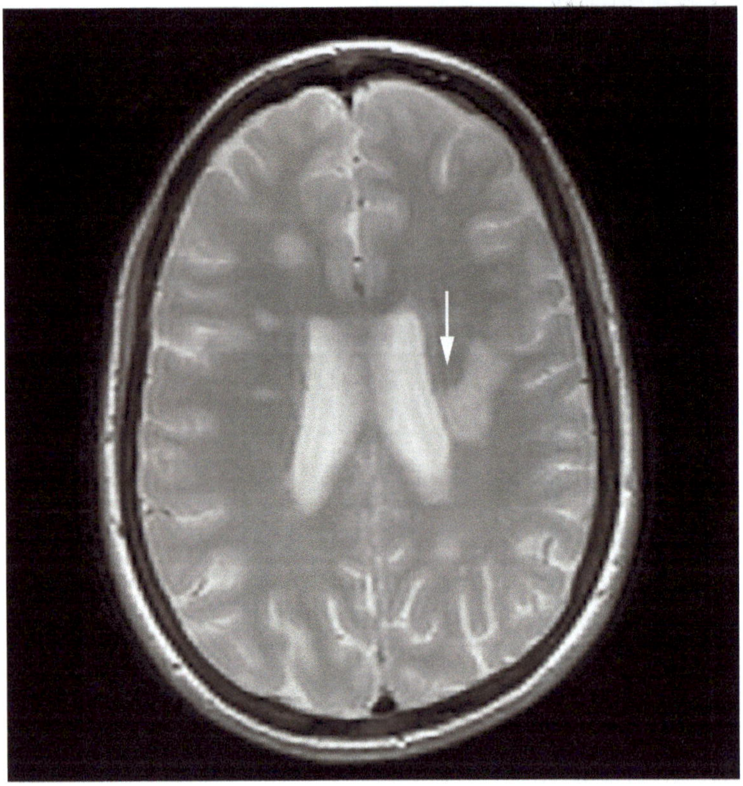

Fig. 1.41 Axial PD image of a patient with MS demonstrates several typical lesions, but one of the lesions has an atypical shape and extends from the periventricular to the juxtacortical region (*arrow*)

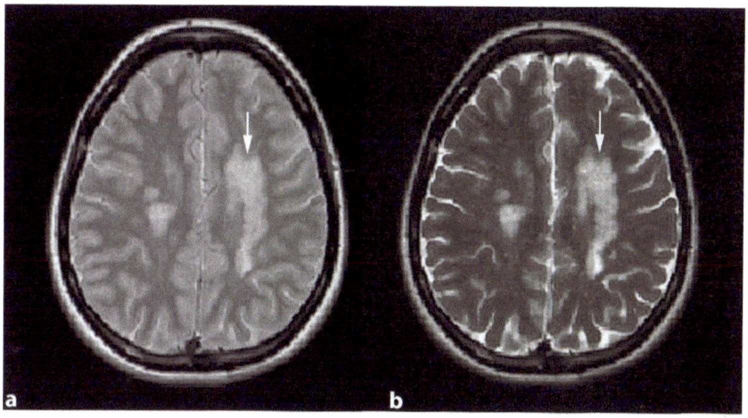

Fig. 1.42 Axial PD- (**a**) and T2-weighted (**b**) images of a patient with MS demonstrate a large confluent lesion (*arrows*). The lesion has no space-occupying effect

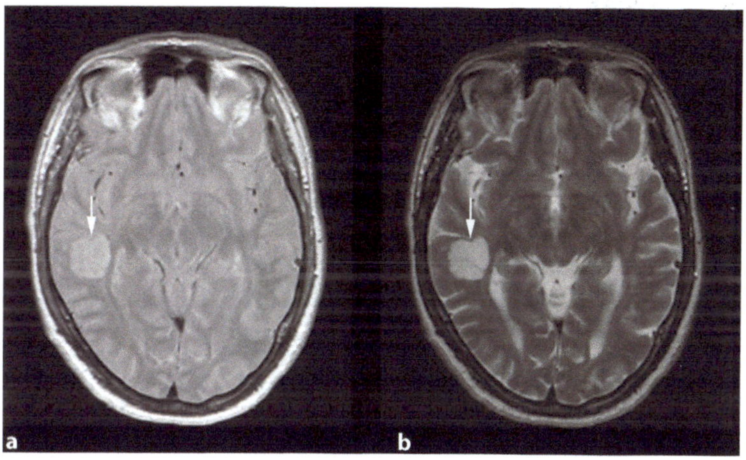

Fig. 1.43 Axial PD- (**a**) and T2-weighted (**b**) images of a patient with MS demonstrate a large temporal lesion (*arrows*)

1.6 Atypical Lesions

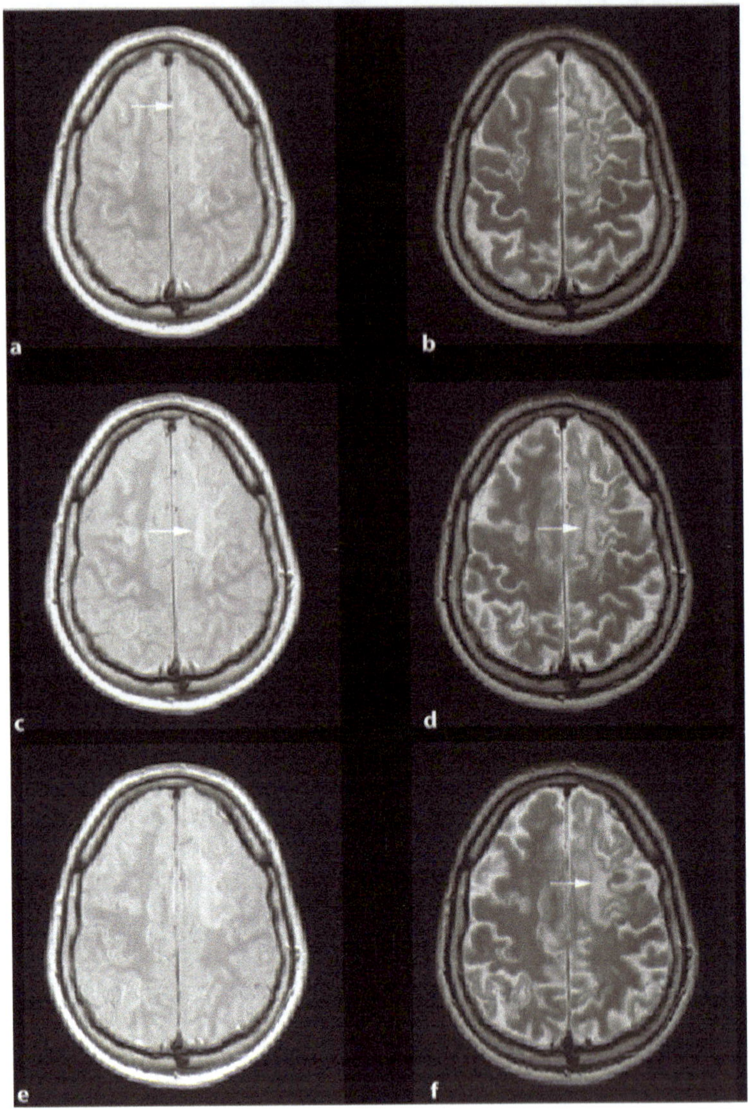

Fig. 1.44 Axial PD- (**a,c,e**) and T2-weighted (**b,d,f**) images of a patient with MS demonstrate a large atypical lesion in the right frontal lobe extending to the parietal lobe (*arrows*)

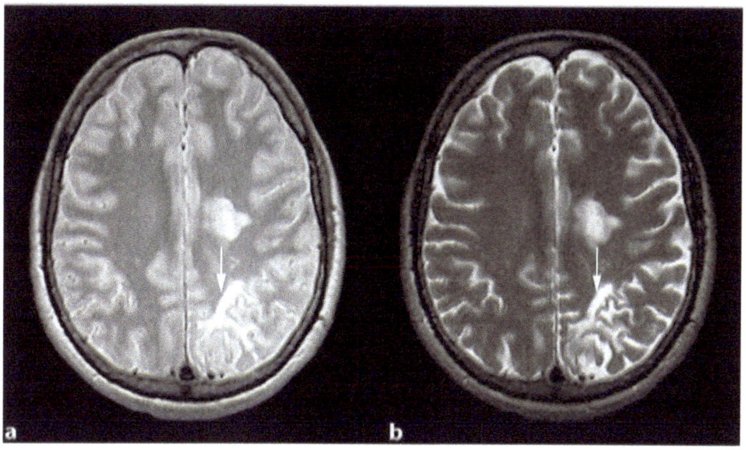

Fig. 1.45 Axial PD- (**a**) and T2-weighted (**b**) images of a patient with RRMS demonstrate an atypical subcortical lesion (*arrows*)

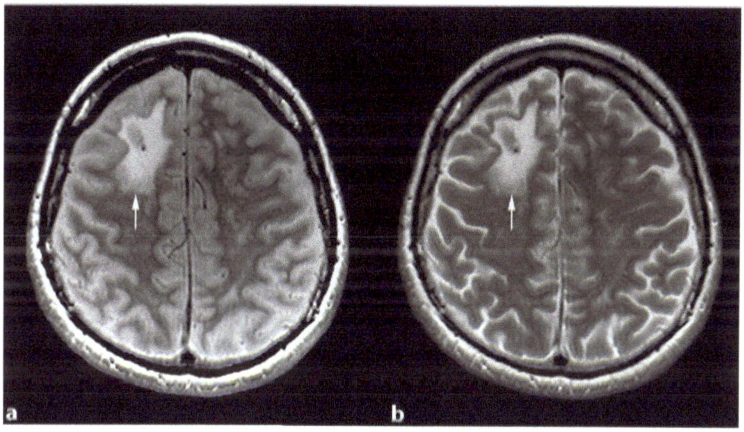

Fig. 1.46 Axial PD- (**a**) and T2-weighted (**b**) images of a patient with MS demonstrate a large atypical lesion in the right frontal lobe (*arrows*). Central isointensity is due to tissue changes after biopsy

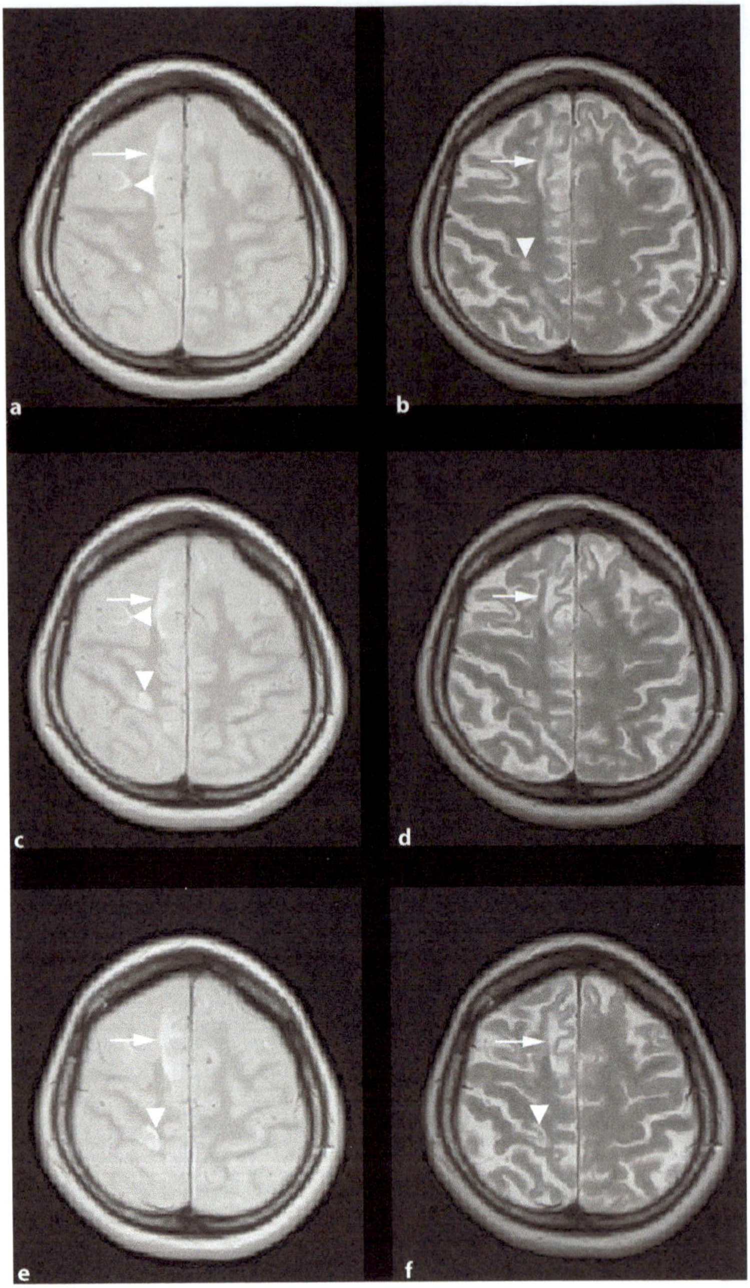

Fig. 1.47 Axial PD- (**a**, **c**, **e**) and T2-weighted consecutive images (**b**, **d**, **f**) of a patient with MS demonstrate an atypical lesion in the right frontal area (*arrows*). Other lesions involving U fibers are demonstrated by *arrowheads*. Special attention should be given to this kind of atypical lesions in patients who receive medication evoking progressive multifocal leukoencephalopathy (PML)

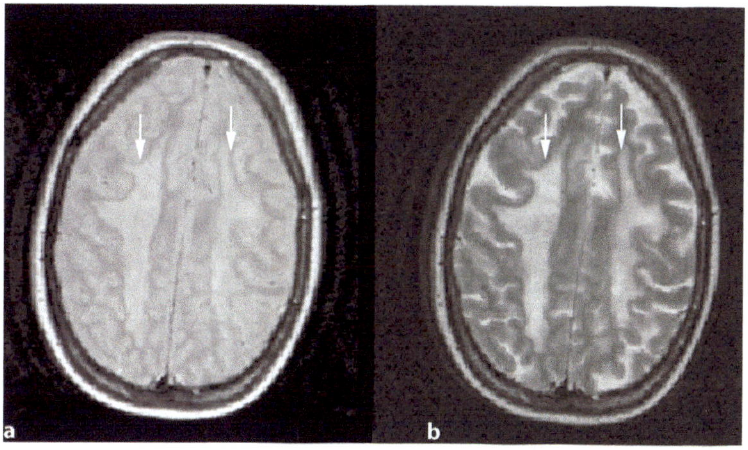

Fig. 1.48 Axial PD- (**a**) and T2-weighted (**b**) images of a patient with MS demonstrate bilateral atypical, more or less symmetric large lesions extending from frontal to parieto-occipital lobes (*arrows*). Note: If such atypical lesions are found, special attention should be given to the diagnosis and other possible differential diagnoses should be clinically excluded

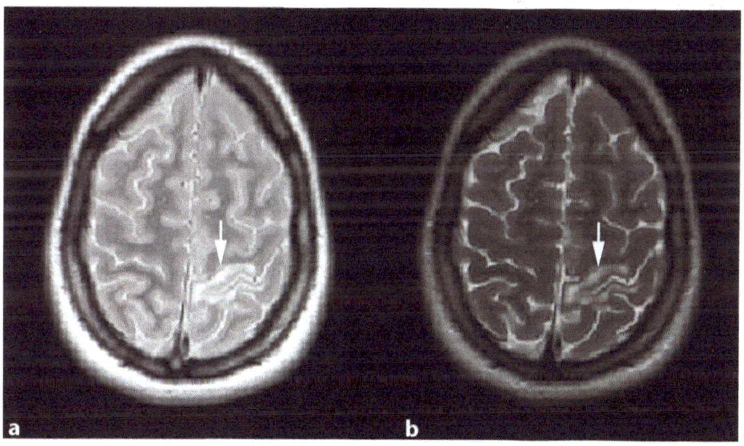

Fig. 1.49 Axial PD- (**a**) and T2-weighted (**b**) images demonstrate an atypical juxtacortical lesion (*arrows*)

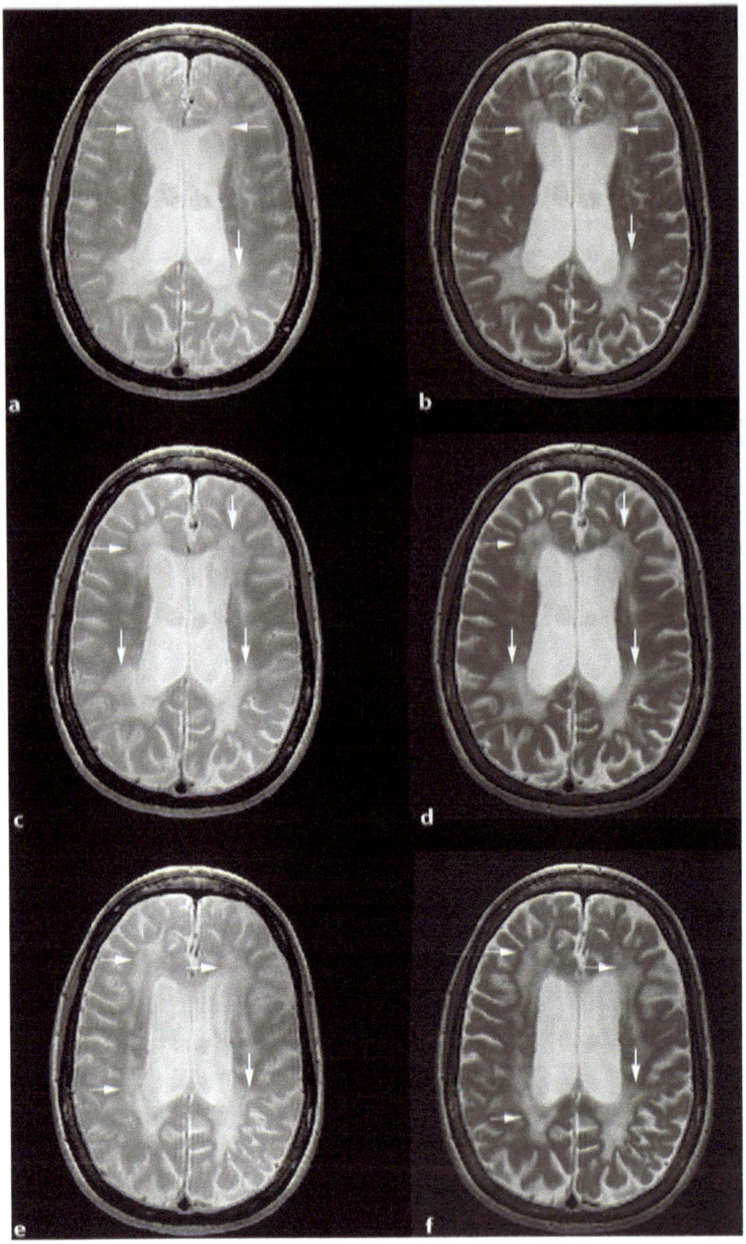

Fig. 1.50 Axial PD- (**a,c,e**) and T2-weighted (**b,d,f**) consecutive images of a patient with secondary progressive MS (SPMS) demonstrate a large volume of T2 lesions and several confluent lesions around the ventricles (*arrows*). Note: Patients with the secondary progressive type of the disease have more confluent plaques and larger volume of T2 lesions, compared with patients with RRMS. In this case, a clear distinction should be made from the dirty white matter

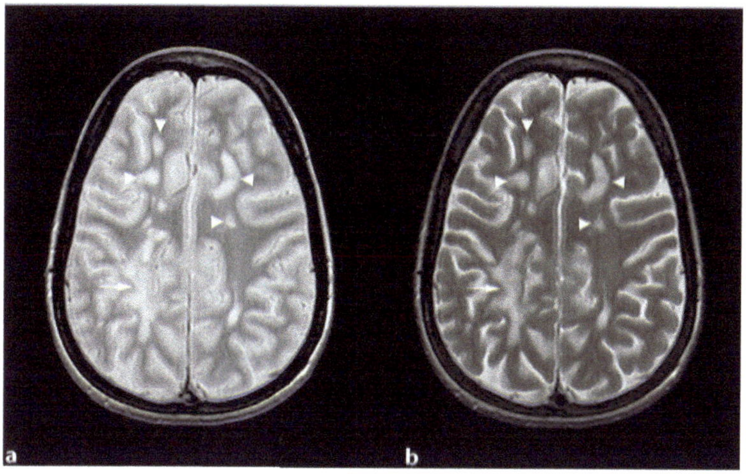

Fig. 1.51 Axial PD- (a) and T2-weighted (**b**) images of a patient with MS demonstrate an atypical lesion in the left parietal lobe (*arrows*) and several typical lesions (*arrowheads*). Note: The presence of typical lesions helps in diagnosing MS. Appearance of such a large atypical lesion may be due to MS per se, but concomitant pathologies should also be considered in special cases

References

1. Barkhof F (1999) MRI in multiple sclerosis: correlation with expanded disability status scale (EDSS). Mult Scler 5:283–286
2. Brownell B, Hughes JT (1962) The distribution of plaques in the cerebrum in multiple sclerosis. J Neurol Neurosurg Psychiatry 25:315–320
3. Bruck W, Bitsch A, Kolenda H et al (1997) Inflammatory central nervous system demyelination: correlation of magnetic resonance imaging findings with lesion pathology. Ann Neurol 42:783–793
4. Ciccarelli O, Werring DJ, Wheeler-Kingshott CA et al (2001) Investigation of MS normal-appearing brain using diffusion tensor MRI with clinical correlations. Neurology 56:926–933
5. De Groot CJ, Bergers E, Kamphorst W et al (2001) Post-mortem MRI-guided sampling of multiple sclerosis brain lesions: increased yield of active demyelinating and (p) reactive lesions. Brain 124:1635–1645
6. De Stefano N, Narayanan S, Francis SJ et al (2002) Diffuse axonal and tissue injury in patients with multiple sclerosis with low cerebral lesion load and no disability. Arch Neurol 59:1565–1571
7. Ge Y (2006) Multiple sclerosis: the role of MR imaging. AJNR Am J Neuroradiol 27:1165–1176
8. Goodin DS (2006) Magnetic resonance imaging as a surrogate outcome measure of disability in multiple sclerosis: have we been overly harsh in our assessment? Ann Neurol 59:597–605
9. Kidd D, Barkhof F, McConnell R et al (1999) Cortical lesions in multiple sclerosis. Brain 122:17–26
10. O'Riordan JI, Thompson AJ, Kingsley DP et al (1998) The prognostic value of brain MRI

in clinically isolated syndromes of the CNS: a 10-year follow-up. Brain 121:495–503
11. Ormerod IE, Miller DH, McDonald WI et al (1987) The role of NMR imaging in the assessment of multiple sclerosis and isolated neurological lesions: a quantitative study. Brain 110:1579–1616
12. Ostuni JL, Richert ND, Lewis BK et al (1999) Characterization of differences between multiple sclerosis and normal brain: a global magnetization transfer application. AJNR Am J Neuroradiol 20:501–507
13. Paty DW (1998) Magnetic resonance imaging in the assessment of disease activity in multiple sclerosis. Can J Neurol Sci 15:266–272
14. Peterson JW, Bo L, Mork S et al (2001) Transected neurites, apoptotic neurons, and reduced inflammation in cortical multiple sclerosis lesions. Ann Neurol 50:389–400
15. Rovaris M, Comi G, Ladkani D et al (2003) Short-term correlations between clinical and MR imaging findings in relapsing-remitting multiple sclerosis. AJNR Am J Neuroradiol 24:75–81
16. Simon JH, Li D, Traboulsee A et al (2006) Standardized MR imaging protocol for multiple sclerosis: Consortium of MS Centers consensus guidelines. AJNR Am J Neuroradiol 27:455–461
17. Smith ME, Stone LA, Albert PS et al (1993) Clinical worsening in multiple sclerosis is associated with increased frequency and area of gadopentetate dimeglumine-enhancing magnetic resonance imaging lesions. Ann Neurol 33:480–489
18. Stewart WA, Hall LD, Berry K et al (1984) Correlation between NMR scan and brain slice data in multiple sclerosis. Lancet 2:412
19. Thorpe JW, Kidd D, Moseley IF et al (1996) Serial gadolinium-enhanced MRI of the brain and spinal cord in early relapsing-remitting multiple sclerosis. Neurology 46:373–378
20. Zhao GJ, Koopmans RA, Li DK et al (2000) Effect of interferon beta-1b in MS: assessment of annual accumulation of proton density (PD)/T2 activity on MRI. UBC MS/MRI Analysis Group and the MS Study Group. Neurology 11:200–206

2 MS Lesions in Fluid Attenuated Inversion Recovery Images

M.A. Sahraian, E.-W. Radue

2.1 Introduction

Fluid attenuated inversion recovery (FLAIR) MR sequences produce heavily T2-weighted images by nulling the signal from cerebrospinal fluid (CSF), using an inversion time that usually ranges from 1,800 to 2,500 ms (Adams and Melhem 1999). By suppressing the signal intensity of bulk water, FLAIR images increase the conspicuousness of lesions located in the periventricular area. Tissue water is also affected, therefore FLAIR images provide a better lesion contrast than do PD- or T2-weighted images, particularly in gray matter (up to 30%, Yousry et al.). This technique was first reported by Hajnal et al. (1992). Because of its unique characteristics in identifying lesions close to the ventricles, juxtacortical, and especially cortical regions, it has attracted strong attention of radiologists for its clinical utility. Unfortunately, FLAIR images are less sensitive in the depiction of lesions involving brainstem and cerebellum, so lesion load may be underestimated in the posterior fossa (Gawne-Cain et al. 1998). Two other disadvantages of FLAIR MR sequences are CSF flow artifacts and the long acquisition time required for imaging an only limited number of slices. Pulsatile CSF flow generates inflow effects in the selected slice during the inversion time interval, which causes incomplete nulling of CSF signal intensities, and may produce hyperintense artifacts in areas of prominent CSF pulsation, like the foramen of Monro and third and fourth ventricles (Bakshi et al. 2000). The limitation of long acquisition time has been overcome by applying fast spin-echo images (Rydberg et al. 1994). The quality of spinal FLAIR imaging is variable and often degraded by motion artifacts arising from CSF pulsation. Although FLAIR can produce visually pleasing images of the spinal cord, it is less sensitive in the detection of lesions than T2-weighted images are (Castillo et al. 2000). Looking at the output data it is concluded that FLAIR can be added to the examination of a patient suspected for MS or in established MS, but it should not substitute other sequences such as PD-weighted images.

2.2 Location, Shape and Size

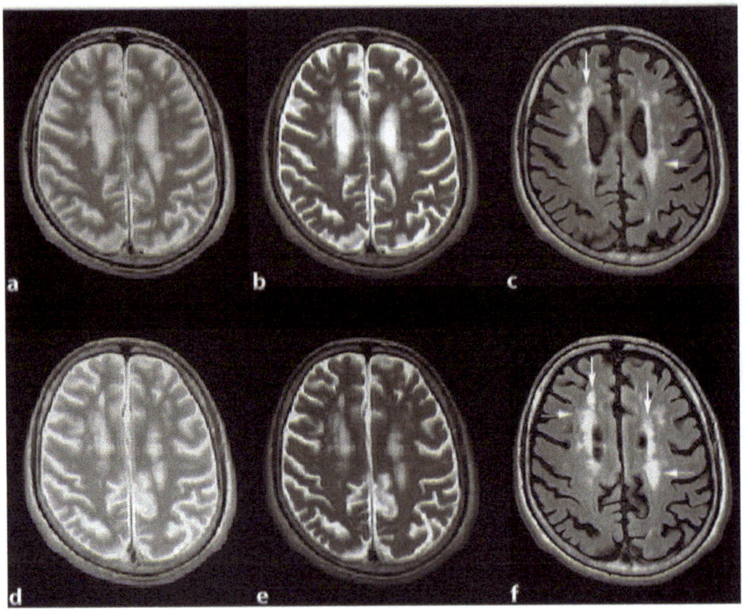

Fig. 2.1 Axial PD (**a,d**), T2-weighted (**b,e**), and FLAIR (**c,f**) consecutive images of a patient with MS demonstrate multiple hyperintense lesions around the lateral ventricles (*arrows*). Note: Periventricular lesions are best depicted by FLAIR images due to suppression of CSF signal and high signal difference between CSF and lesions

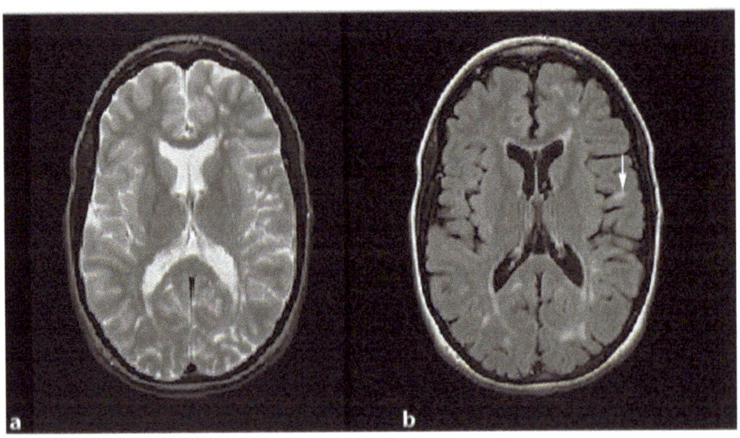

Fig. 2.2 Axial T2-weighted (**a**) and FLAIR (**b**) images demonstrate a lesion in the cortical and juxtacortical area (*arrow*). Note: Lesions in the juxtacortical area are better detected on FLAIR images

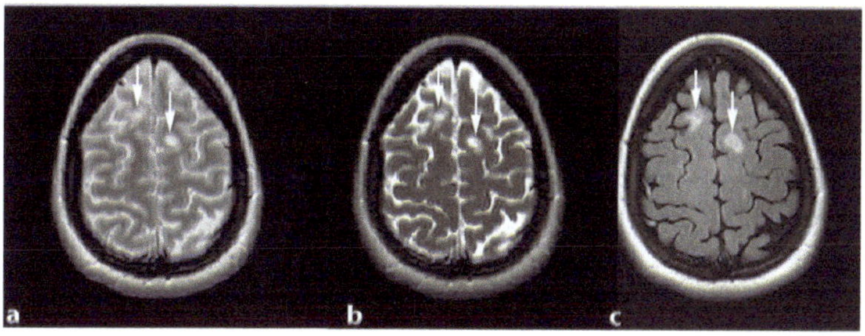

Fig. 2.3 Axial PD- (**a**), T2-weighted (**b**), and FLAIR (**c**) images of a patient with MS demonstrate two lesions involving cortex and the juxtacortical area (*arrows*)

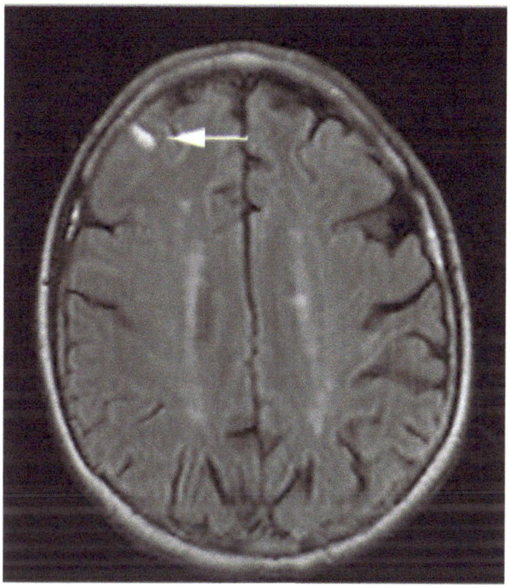

Fig. 2.4 Axial FLAIR image of a patient with MS demonstrates a cortical lesion (*arrow*)

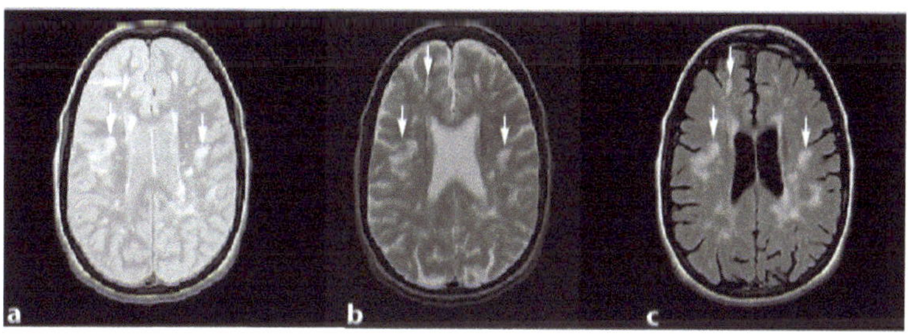

Fig. 2.5 Axial PD- (**a**), T2-weighted (**b**), and FLAIR (**c**) images demonstrate superiority of FLAIR in detecting juxtacortical lesions (*arrows*)

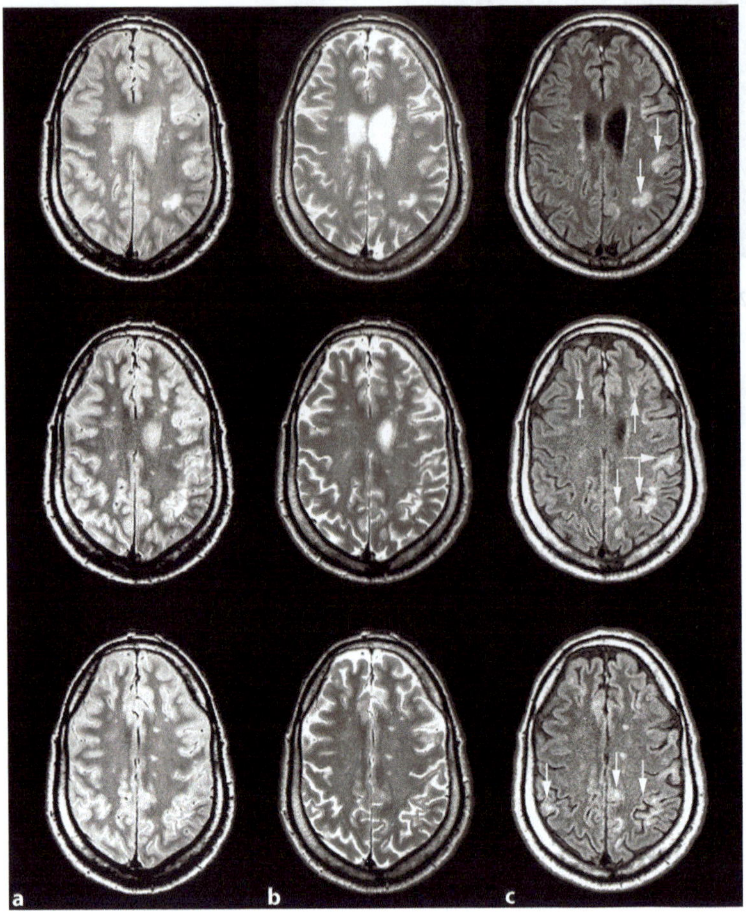

Fig. 2.6 Axial consecutive PD- (**a**), T2-weighted (**b**), and FLAIR (**c**) images of a patient with MS demonstrate typical juxtacortical lesions that touch the cortex and are better depicted on FLAIR sequence (*arrows*)

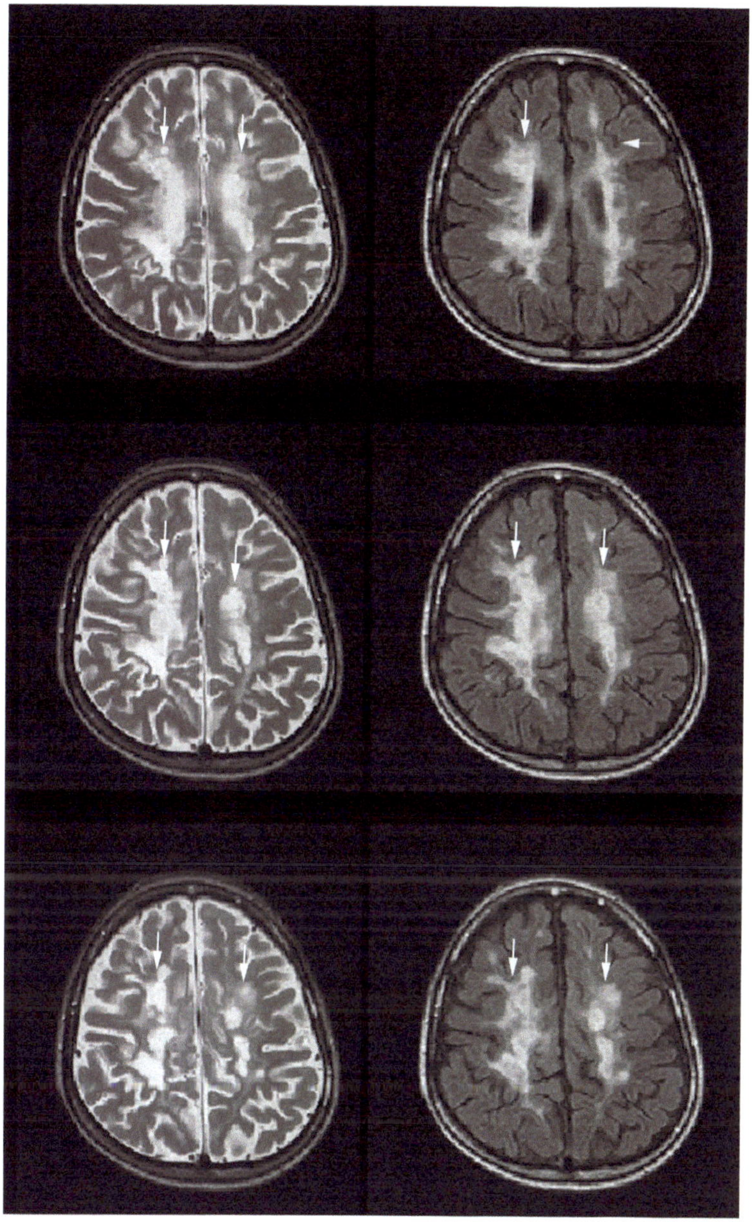

Fig. 2.7 Axial T2-weighted (*left column*) and FLAIR (*right column*) images of a patient with MS demonstrate confluent periventricular lesions (*arrows*). Note: The borders of lesions and CSF may be not clear in T2-weighted images, but FLAIR can demonstrate the boundaries of the ventricles better than can the other sequences. The differentiation between CSF and lesions is easily possible

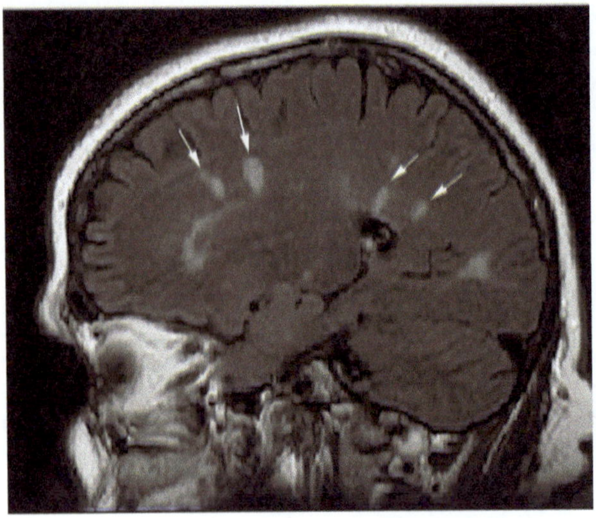

Fig. 2.8 Sagittal FLAIR image of a patient with MS demonstrates ovoid lesions perpendicular to the surface of the ventricles. This type of lesions in sagittal images is typical for MS

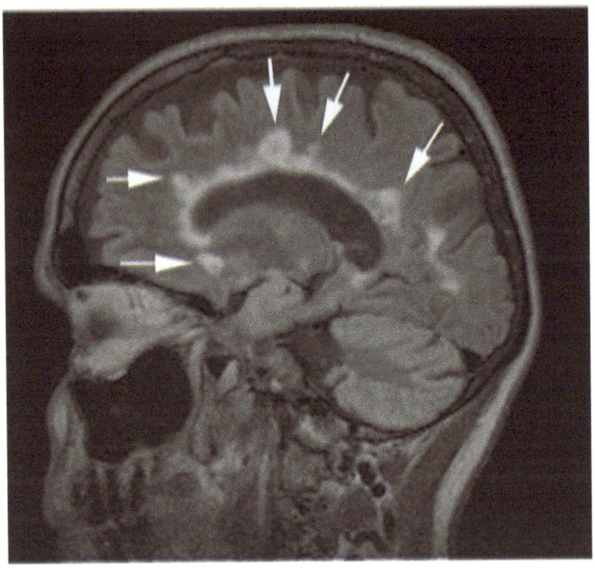

Fig. 2.9 Sagittal FLAIR image of a patient with MS demonstrates ovoid lesions perpendicular to the ventricular surface (Dawson's fingers) (*arrows*). Note: Dawson's fingers refer to the oval, elongated lesions in the corona radiata and the centrum semiovale. These lesions are orientated along the subependymal veins that are perpendicular to the walls of the ventricles and are best demonstrated in sagittal FLAIR images

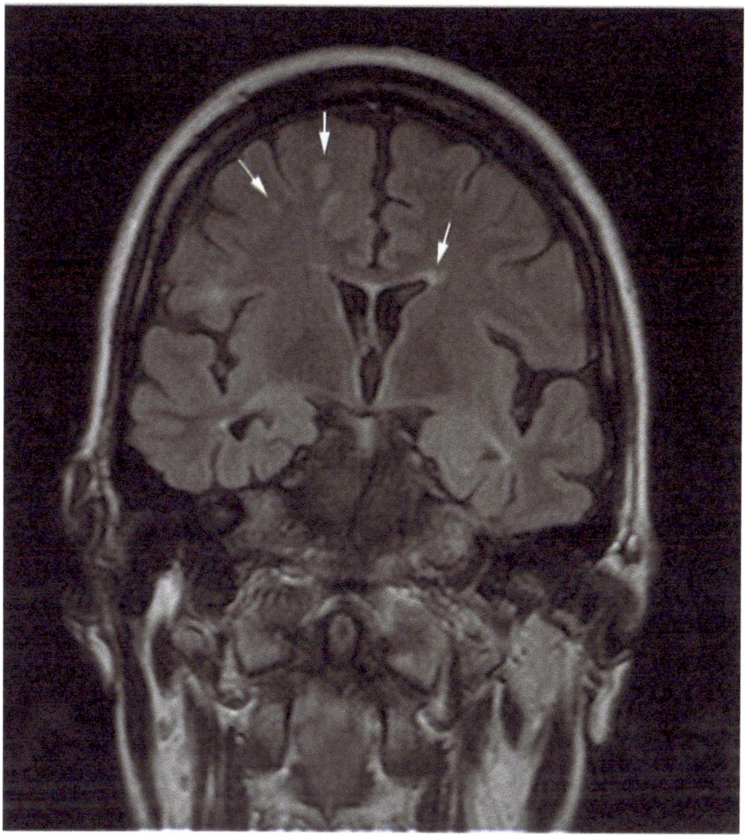

Fig. 2.10 Coronal FLAIR image of a patient with MS demonstrates several hyperintense lesions (*arrows*)

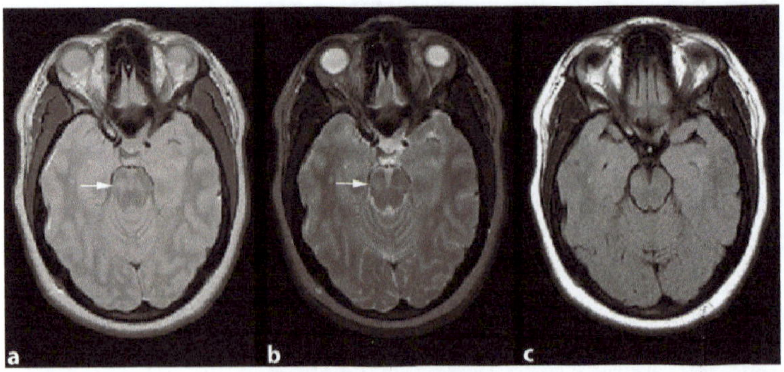

Fig. 2.11 Axial PD- (a), T2-weighted (**b**), and FLAIR (**c**) images of a patient with RRMS demonstrate a pontine lesion (*arrows*) that is not demonstrated on the FLAIR sequence. Note: Infratentorial lesions are better seen on PD-weighted images than on FLAIR

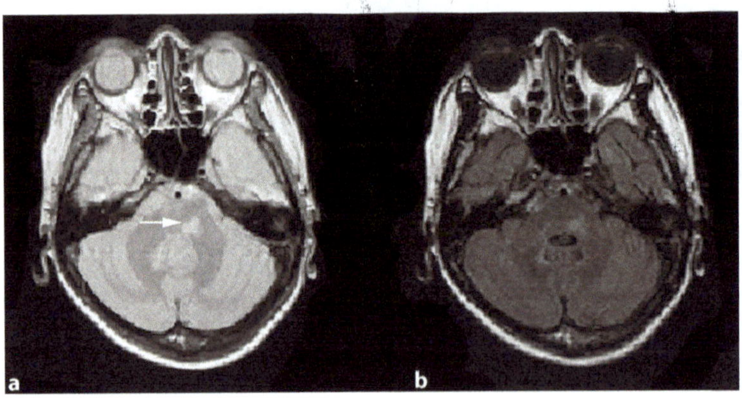

Fig. 2.12 Axial PD (a) and FLAIR (**b**) images demonstrate a lesion attached to the 4th ventricle (*arrows*). The lesion is more prominent on the PD than on the FLAIR sequence

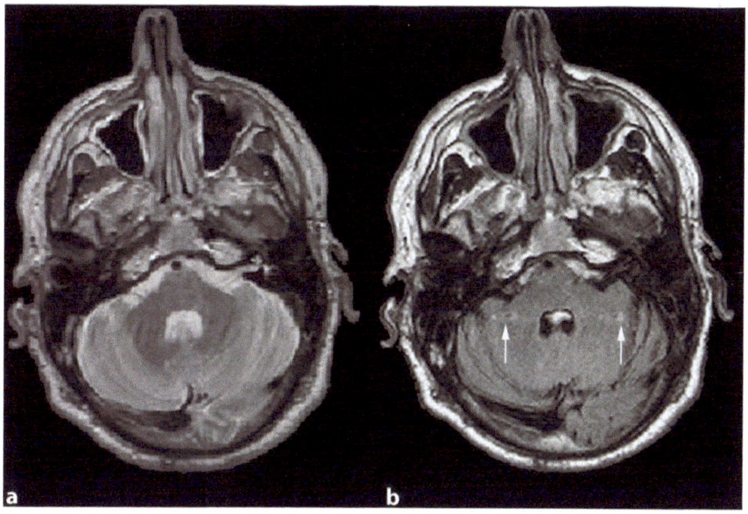

Fig. 2.13 Axial PD (**a**) and FLAIR (**b**) images demonstrate two flow artifacts, hyperintense on FLAIR in the cerebellar peduncle (*arrows*). Note: FLAIR sequences may induce more artifacts than do PD images, especially in the posterior fossa and the ventricles

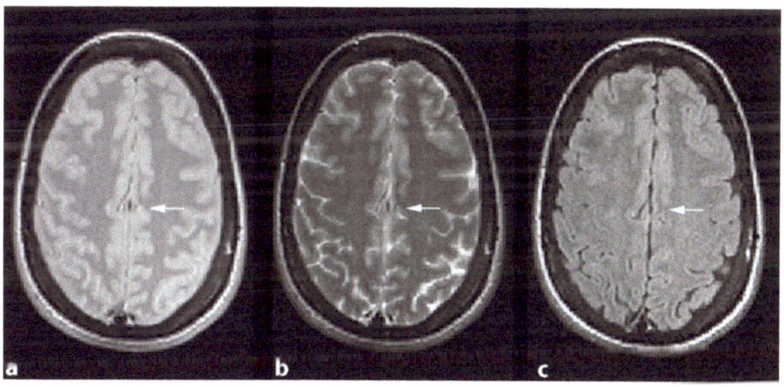

Fig. 2.14 Axial PD- (**a**) and T2-weighted (**b**) images demonstrate a hyperintense area that is hypointense on FLAIR (**c**) (*arrows*). Note: FLAIR images can help in differentiating normal structures and other pathologies like small cysts from MS lesions

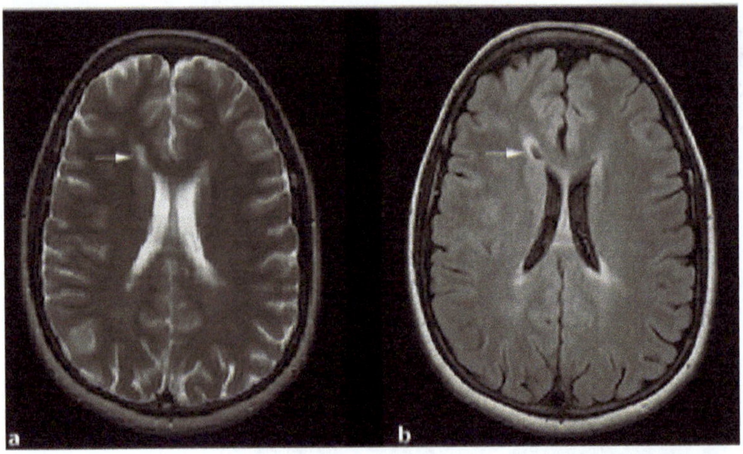

Fig. 2.15 Axial PD (**a**) and FLAIR (**b**) images of a patient with MS demonstrate periventricular lesions (*arrows*). Note: The hyperintensity that has been demonstrated on the T2-weighted image by *arrow* may be completely detected as lesion, but comparison with the FLAIR sequence shows that this hyperintensity consists of a lesion and a small part of the ventricle

References

1. Adams JG, Melhem ER (1999) Clinical usefulness of T2-weighted fluid-attenuated inversion recovery MR imaging of the CNS. AJR Am J Roentgenol 172:529–536
2. Bakshi R, Caruthers SD, Janardhan V et al (2000) Intraventricular CSF pulsation artifact on fast fluid-attenuated inversion-recovery MR images: analysis of 100 consecutive normal studies. AJNR Am J Neuroradiol 21:503–508
3. Castillo M, Mukherji SK (2000) Clinical applications of FLAIR, HASTE, and magnetization transfer in neuroimaging. Semin Ultrasound CT MR. 21:417–427
4. Gawne-Cain ML, O'Riordan JI, Coles A et al (1998) MRI lesion volume measurement in multiple sclerosis and its correlation with disability: a comparison of fast fluid attenuated inversion recovery (fFLAIR) and spin echo sequences. J Neurol Neurosurg Psychiatry 64:197–203
5. Hajnal JV, De Coene B, Lewis PD et al (1992) High signal regions in normal white matter shown by heavily T2-weighted CSF nulled IR sequences. J Comput Assist Tomogr 16:506–513
6. Rydberg JN, Hammond CA, Grimm RC et al (1994) Initial clinical experience in MR imaging of the brain with a fast fluid-attenuated inversion-recovery pulse sequence. Radiology 193:173–180

3 Gadolinium Enhancing Lesions in Multiple Sclerosis

M.A. Sahraian, E.-W. Radue

3.1 Introduction

Contrast-enhanced MR imaging is a sensitive method for detecting active MS lesions. Gadolinium (Gd) enhancement is a marker for blood-brain barrier breakdown and histologically correlates with the inflammatory phase of lesion development.

In MS, most new lesions go through a phase of enhancement that usually persists for 2–6 weeks. Only a small number of lesions demonstrates enhancement for 3–4 months (Filppi et al. 2001). Very rarely, plaques may enhance for more than 6 months (He et al. 2001). The natural history of contrast enhancing lesions is highly variable and unpredictable. Among the possible evolutions, axonal loss and axonal degeneration are thought to contribute to clinical worsening and disability (Miller et al. 1998).

Approximately 80% of contrast enhancing lesions appear hypointense on the correlating unenhanced T1-weighted images. However, once contrast enhancement fades, the hypointense lesions may become isointense, and less than 40% of them develop into persistent black holes (van Waesberghe et al. 1998).

This return to the T1 isointense state or mild T1 hypointensity may indicate resolution of edema or partial remyelination.

Enhancing lesions may differ in size, shape, or pattern. Most of them (68%) demonstrate a nodular pattern. Twenty-three percent show ring-like enhancement, and 9% have other enhancement patterns (He et al. 2001).

Ring-like enhancement probably arises from recent inflammation at the periphery of an active lesion in which the blood-brain barrier defect has been partially or completely repaired in the center (Bastianello et al. 1990). It is also noted that ongoing activity affects one margin of the plaque, and the remainder is quiescent, which may be a cause of the formation of arc pattern (He et al. 2001). Nodular enhancing lesions tend to differ in size and also to decrease their size over time.

None of these patterns is specific for MS. The only exception might be the "open-ring" sign for differentiating large, tumor-like demyelinating lesions from actual tumors and infections. These lesions create an incomplete ring and typically the open section is orientated toward the gray matter or is adjacent to it (Bitsch and Bruck 2002).

Most Gd enhancing lesions are clinically silent. Thus, MRI has become an important tool for supporting an early and accurate diagnosis of MS in many patients.

Analysis of studies suggests that Gd enhancement is not a marker of later disability or functional impairment in long-term follow up (Kappos et al. 1999). According to the McDonald criteria, contrast enhanced images can be used for early diagnosis of MS. In patients with an isolated neurological event, suggestive of MS, detection of a new Gd enhanced lesion at least 3 months after the onset of initial clinical event demonstrates dissemination in time (Polman et al. 2005) if the lesion is not at the site corresponding to the initial event.

Steroid treatment may strongly suppress appearance of enhancing lesions, whereas larger Gd dosage may increase sensitivity of blood-brain barrier leakage. This could result in reduced pathological specificity because even old and inactive lesions can show faint enhancement (Bitsch and Bruck 2002).

In this chapter we demonstrate different patterns of enhancing lesions in various parts of the brain. Lesion evolution in detail is demonstrated in the next chapter.

3.2 Different Patterns of Enhancement

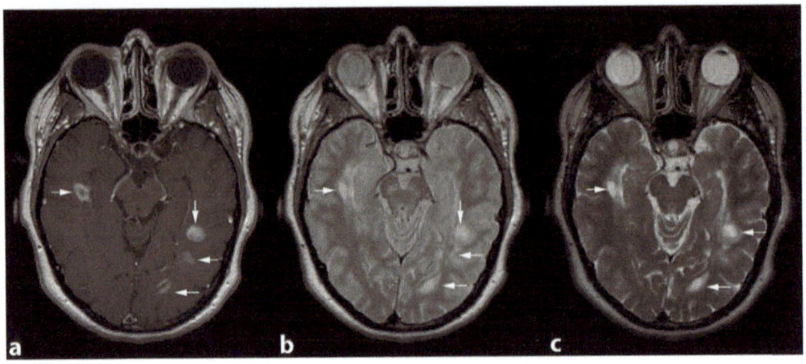

Fig. 3.1 Axial T1-weighted with Gd (**a**), PD- (**b**), and T2-weighted (**c**) images of a patient with RRMS demonstrate several enhancing lesions with corresponding T2-weighted abnormalities (*arrows*). Note: Almost all enhancing lesions have a corresponding T2 abnormality, but in some cases Gd enhancement can precede T2 lesions by hours or days

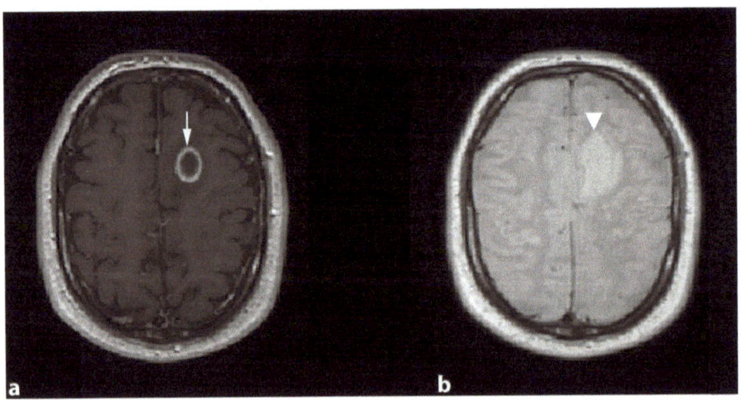

Fig. 3.2 Axial T1-weighted with Gd (**a**) and T2-weighted (**b**) images demonstrate a ring enhancing lesion (*arrow*) and the corresponding T2 hyperintensity (*arrowhead*). Note: Ring enhancing lesions seem to be more destructive, larger, and older than nodular lesions

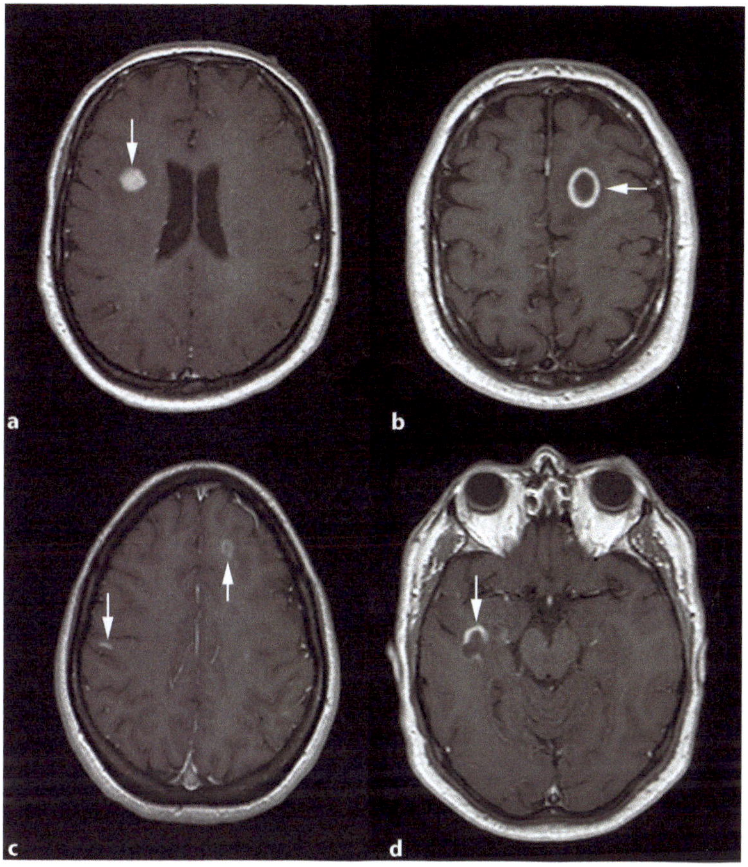

Fig. 3.3 Axial T1-weighted with contrast images of different patients with RRMS demonstrate various patterns of enhancement (*arrows*). Note: Most enhancing lesions are of nodular type with a homogenous pattern of enhancement (**a**), but other patterns like complete ring enhancement (**b**), incomplete ring shape (**d**), or linear shape enhancement (**c**) may be seen in MS

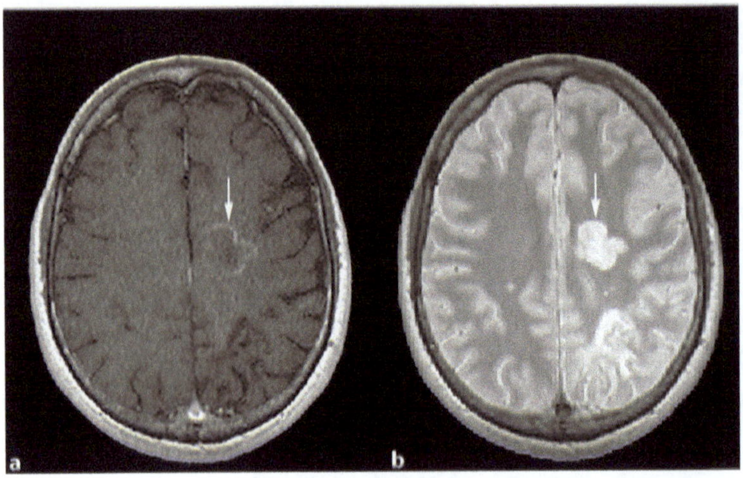

Fig. 3.4 Axial MR image of a patient with MS demonstrates a large lesion on the T2-weighted sequence that has been enhanced in a T1-weighted postcontrast image (*arrow*). Peripheral thin enhancement of the lesion indicates blood-brain barrier impairment at the edges of the lesion

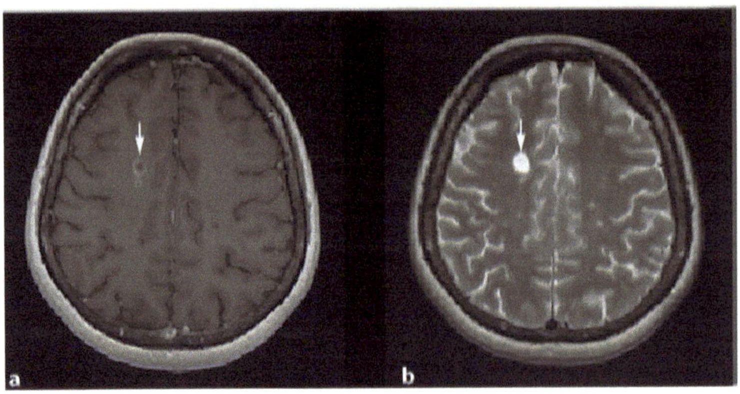

Fig. 3.5 Axial T1-weighted with contrast (a) and T2-weighted (b) images of a patient with RRMS demonstrate two adjacent ring enhancing lesions (*arrows*)

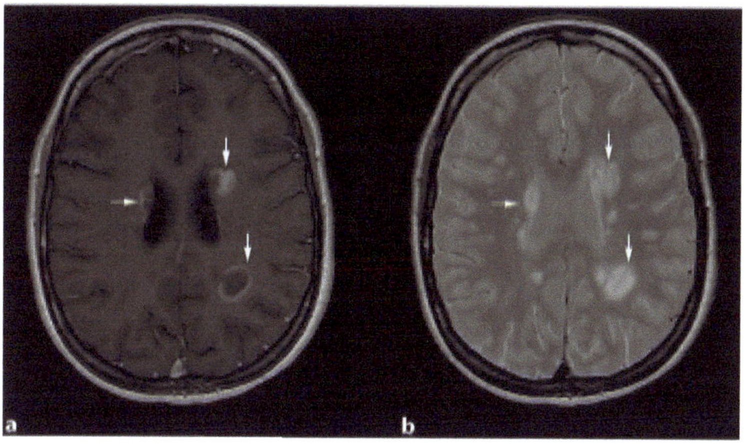

Fig. 3.6 Axial T1-weighted with Gd (**a**) and corresponding PD (**b**) images demonstrate different enhancement patterns in a patient with MS on the same slice (*arrows*)

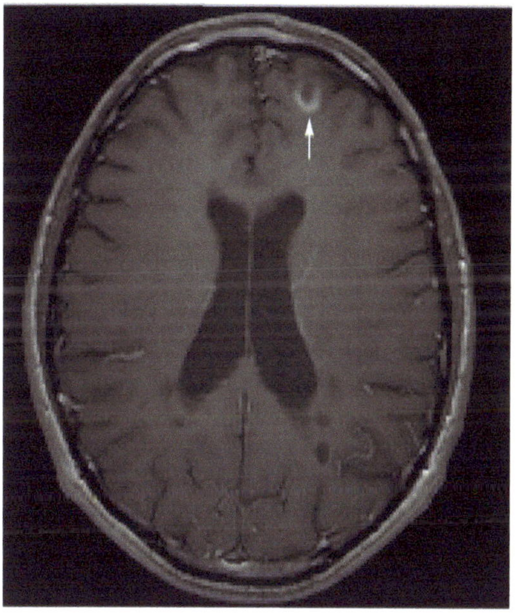

Fig 3.7 Axial T1-weighted image with Gd demonstrates an incomplete ring enhancing lesion in a patient with RRMS (open-ring sign) (*arrow*). Note: An incomplete ring of enhancement that opens where the lesion abuts gray matter may be characteristic for MS

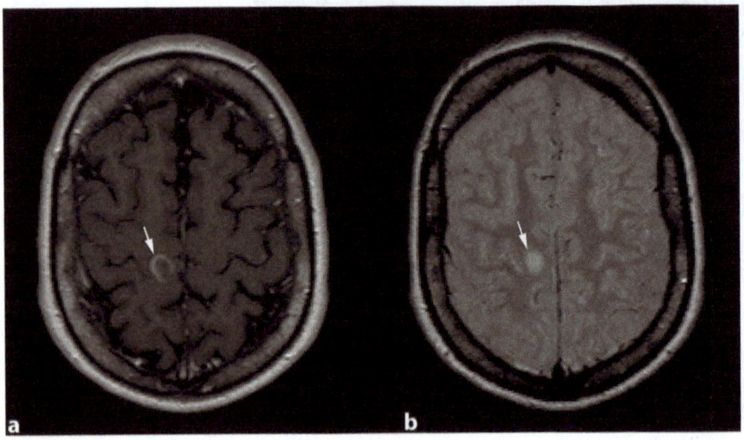

Fig. 3.8 Axial T1-weighted with contrast (**a**) and PD (**b**) images of a patient with MS demonstrate open-ring signs (*arrows*) in the left parietal lobe. Note: Complete ring enhancing lesions pose a common diagnostic challenge and are not valuable in differentiating demyelinating from other pathologies with similar lesions. An open-ring pattern of enhancement is more likely to be associated with demyelinating lesions than are other pathologies

3.3 Shape and Size

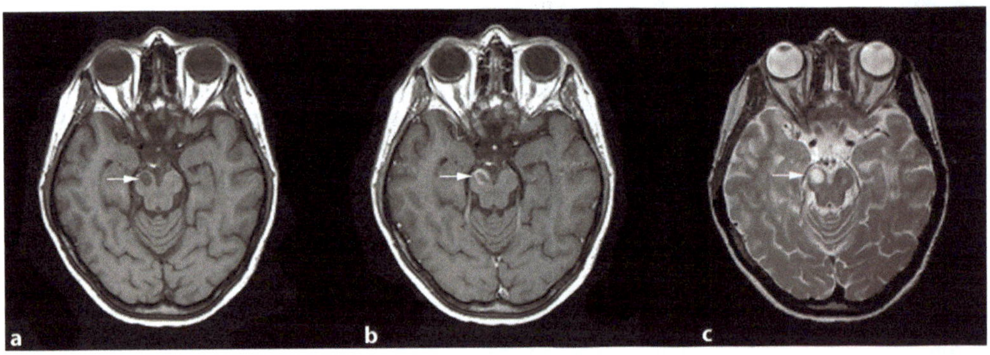

Fig. 3.9 Axial T1-weighted without (**a**), with contrast (**b**), and T2-weighted (**c**) images of a patient with MS demonstrate an incomplete ring enhancing lesion of the midbrain with corresponding hypointensity on T1 without Gd and with T2 hyperintensity (*arrows*)

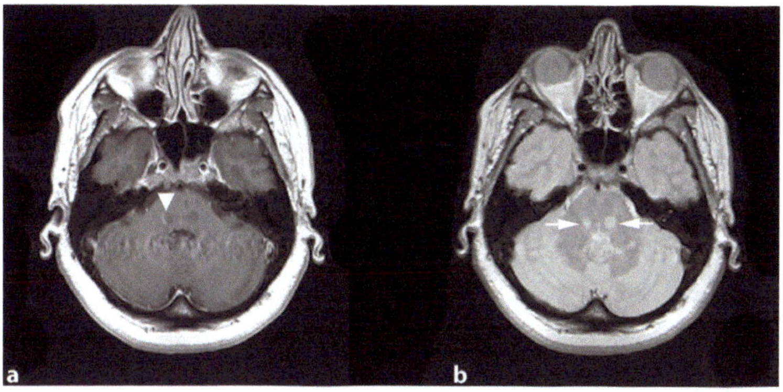

Fig. 3.10 Axial T1-weighted with contrast (**a**) and PD (**b**) images of a patient with RRMS demonstrate two relatively symmetrical lesions in the pons (*arrows*). Note: The lesion on the right side of the pons is partially enhanced (*arrowhead*)

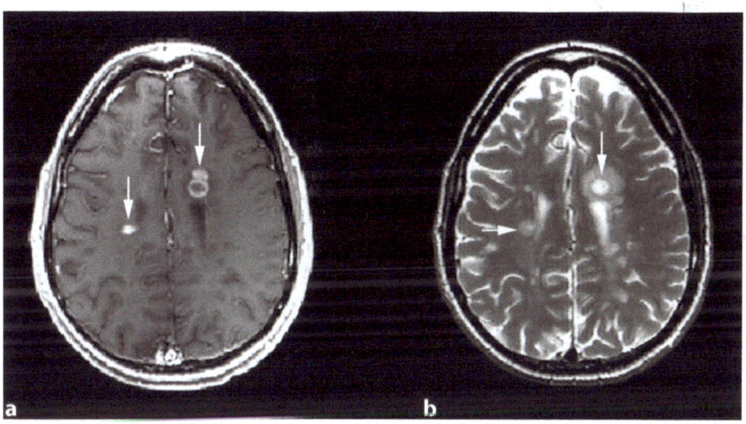

Fig. 3.11 Axial T1-weighted with contrast (**a**) and T2-weighted (**b**) images of a patient with RRMS demonstrate two periventricular enhancing lesions (*arrows*). The enhancing lesion in the left hemisphere demonstrates two separate parts of enhancement

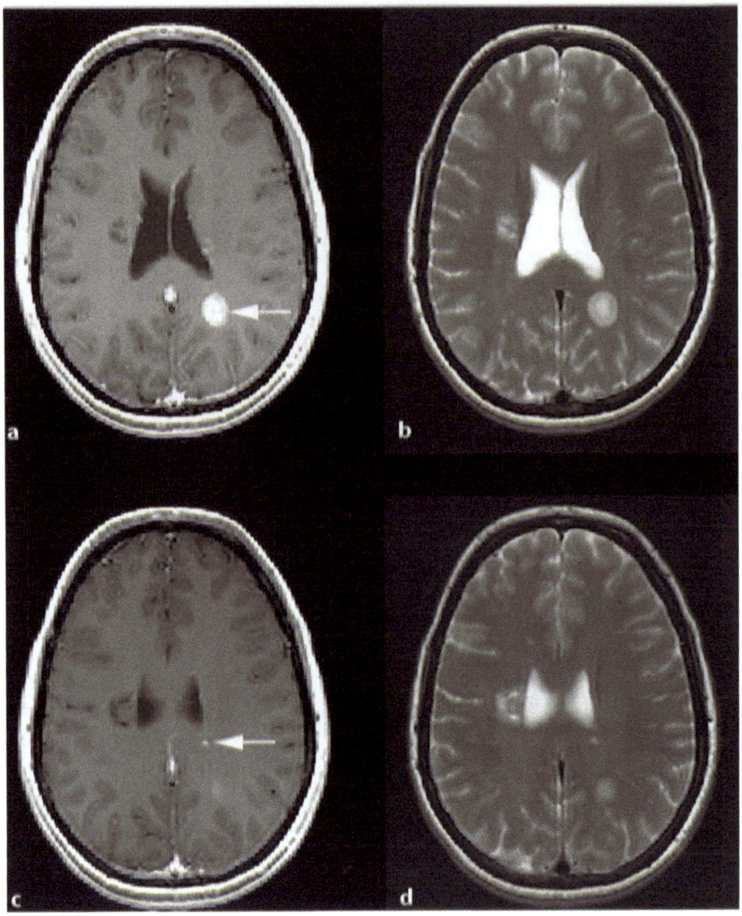

Fig. 3.12 Axial T1-weighted with contrast (**a**,**c**) and corresponding T2-weighted abnormalities (**b**,**d**) of a patient with RRMS demonstrate two enhancing lesions of different sizes at the same time (*arrows*)

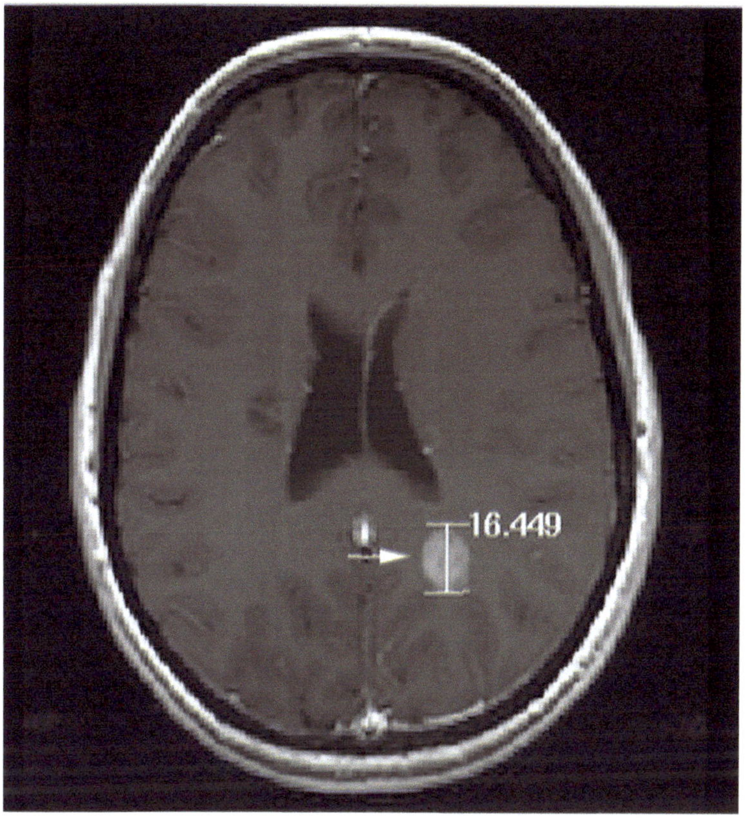

Fig. 3.13 Axial T1-weighted image with contrast demonstrates an enhancing lesion, with measurement of the largest diameter (*arrow*). Note: The size of enhancing lesions differs from a few millimeters to several centimeters, but they are usually small and have little to no mass effect

3.4 Different Locations

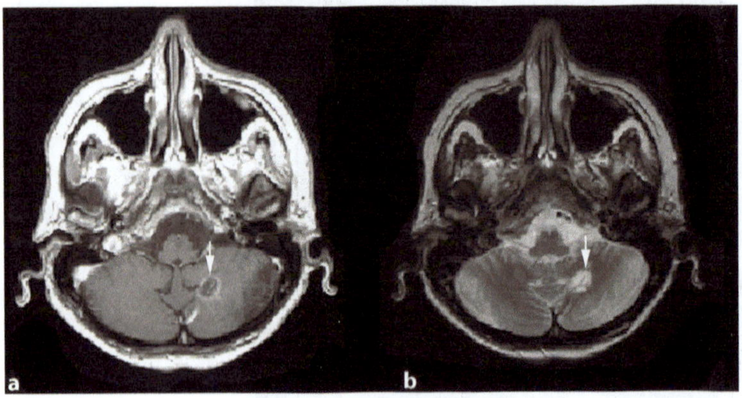

Fig. 3.14 Axial T1-weighted with Gd (**a**) and the corresponding T2-weighted (**b**) images demonstrate a ring enhancing lesion in the cerebellar hemisphere (*arrows*)

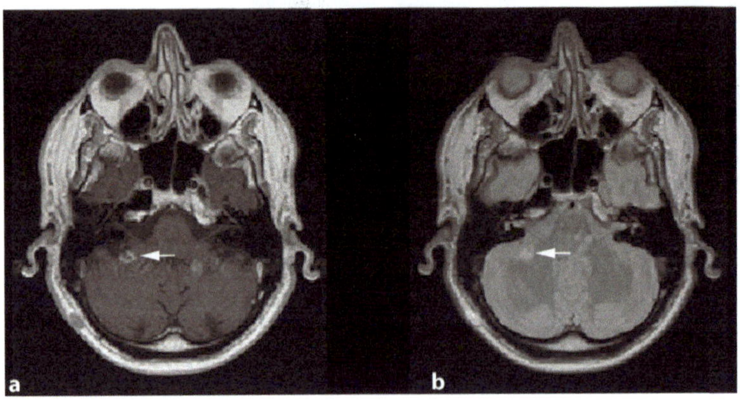

Fig. 3.15 Axial T1-weighted (**a**) with contrast and PD (**b**) images of a patient with RRMS demonstrate an enhancing lesion of the cerebellar peduncle with corresponding PD hyperintensity (*arrows*)

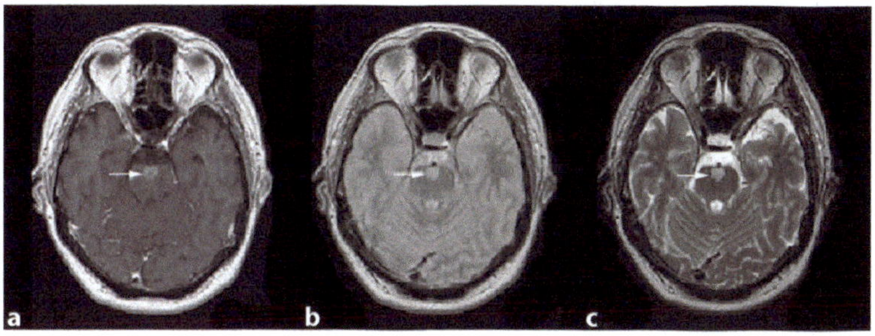

Fig. 3.16 Axial T1-weighted with contrast (**a**), PD- (**b**), and T2-weighted (**c**) images of a patient with RRMS demonstrate an enhancing pontine lesion with corresponding abnormalities (*arrows*)

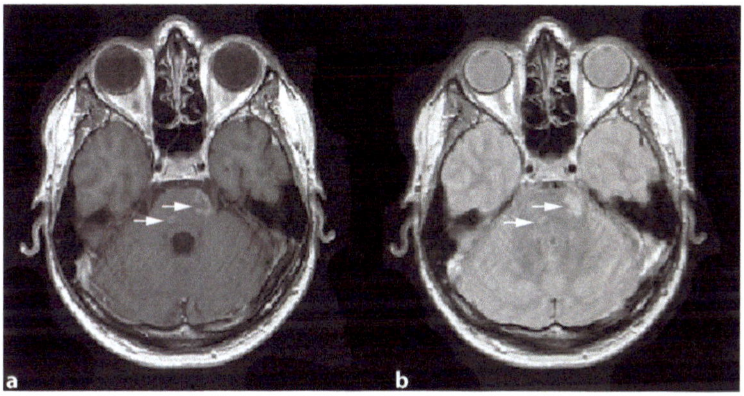

Fig. 3.17 Axial T1-weighted (**a**) with contrast and corresponding PD (**b**) images demonstrate two enhancing lesions in the pons with different patterns (*arrows*)

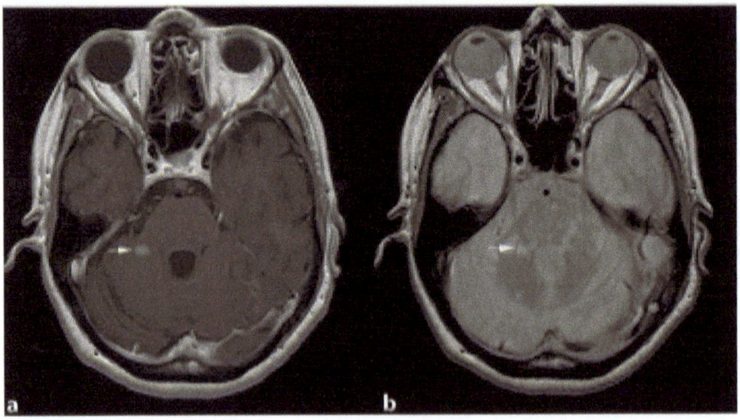

Fig. 3.18 Axial T1-weighted (**a**) with contrast and corresponding PD (**b**) images demonstrate a nodular enhancing lesion of the cerebellar peduncle (*arrows*)

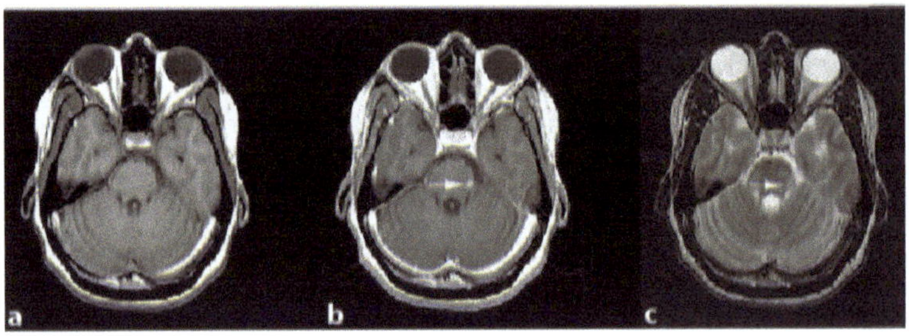

Fig. 3.19 Axial T1 without contrast (**a**) and with contrast (**b**) images of a patient with RRMS demonstrate a small enhancing lesion of the pons with corresponding hyperintensity on the T2 (**c**) image and hypointensity on the T1 image without contrast (*arrows*)

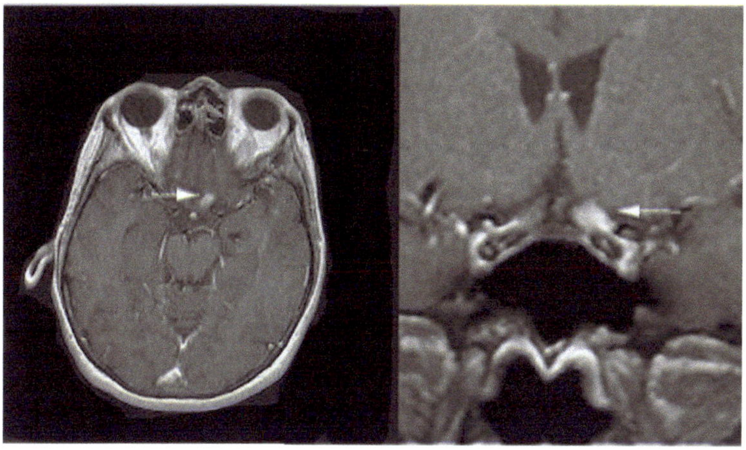

Fig. 3.20 Axial and coronal T1-weighted images with contrast in a patient with optic neuritis demonstrate enhancement of optic chiasma (*arrows*)

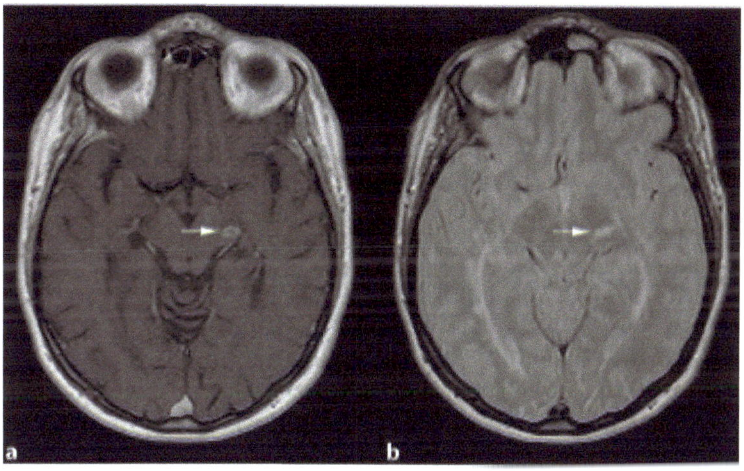

Fig. 3.21 Axial T1-weighted with Gd (a) and corresponding T2-weighted images (b) demonstrate a lesion of the mesencephalon (*arrows*)

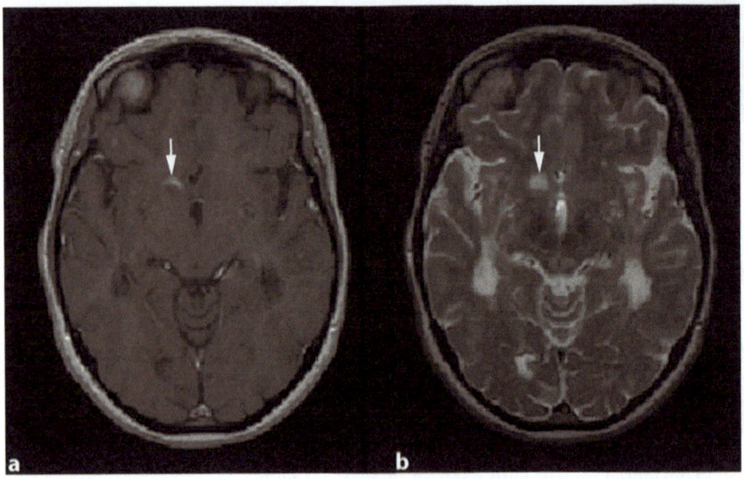

Fig. 3.22 Axial T1-weighted (**a**) with contrast and T2-weighted (**b**) images of a patient with MS demonstrate an enhancing lesion (partial ring) in the base of right frontal lobe (*arrows*)

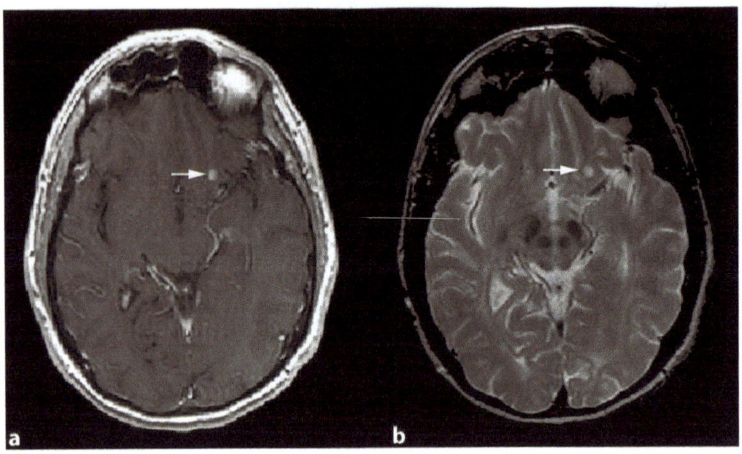

Fig. 3.23 Axial T1-weighted with contrast (**a**) and T2-weighted (**b**) images of a patient with RRMS demonstrate an enhancing lesion in the base of the left frontal lobe near the olfactory nerve (*arrows*)

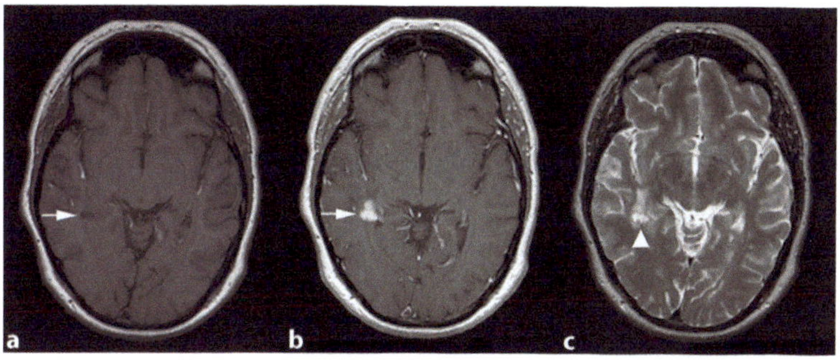

Fig. 3.24 Axial T1-weighted without (**a**) and with Gadolinium (**b**) and T2-weighted images demonstrate an enhancing lesion around the trigone of the lateral ventricle (*arrow*). Look at the corresponding T1 hypointensity (*arrow*) and T2-weighted abnormality (*arrowhead*)

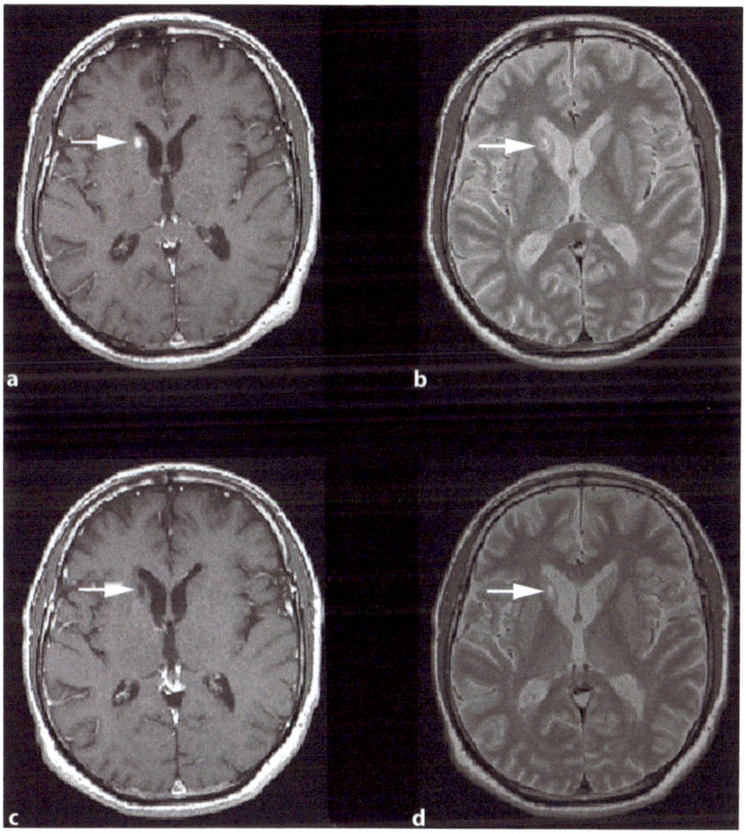

Fig. 3.25 Axial T1-weighted (**a**) with contrast and corresponding T2 (**b**) images demonstrate an enhancing lesion in the caudate nucleus (*arrows*). Follow-up examinations after 1 year (**c,d**) demonstrate that the enhancing lesion has changed into a chronic hypointensity (*arrow*)

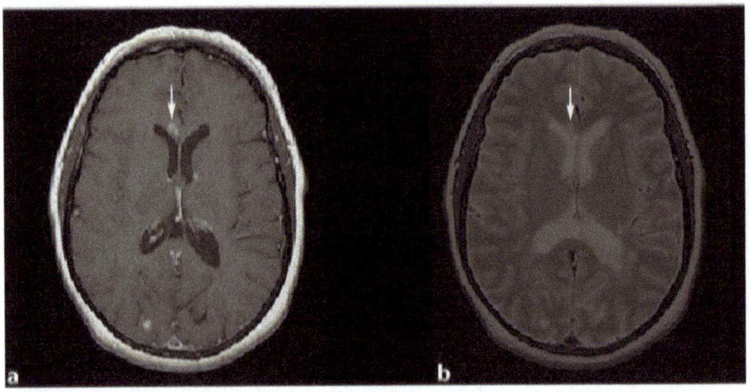

Fig. 3.26 Axial T1-weighted with Gd (**a**) and corresponding T2-weighted (**b**) images of a patient with RRMS demonstrate an enhancing lesion of the genu of the corpus callosum (*arrows*)

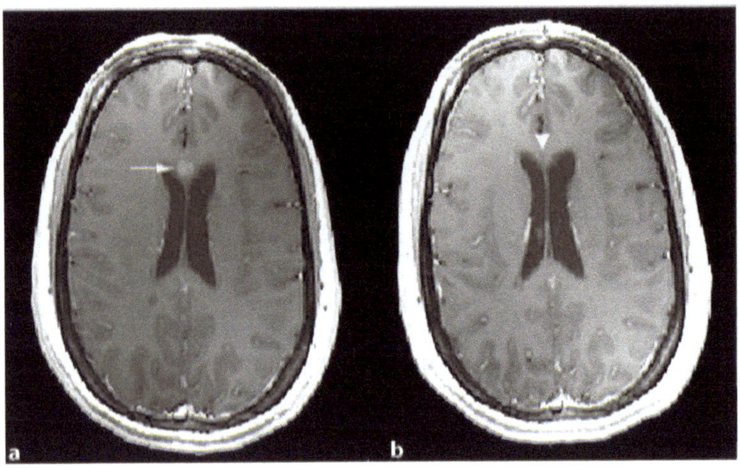

Fig. 3.27 Axial T1-weighted images with contrast at baseline (**a**) and its follow-up after 1 year (**b**) demonstrate an enhancing lesion of the genu of the corpus callosum (*arrow*) that has changed into a isointense lesion with Gd enhancement (*arrowhead*)

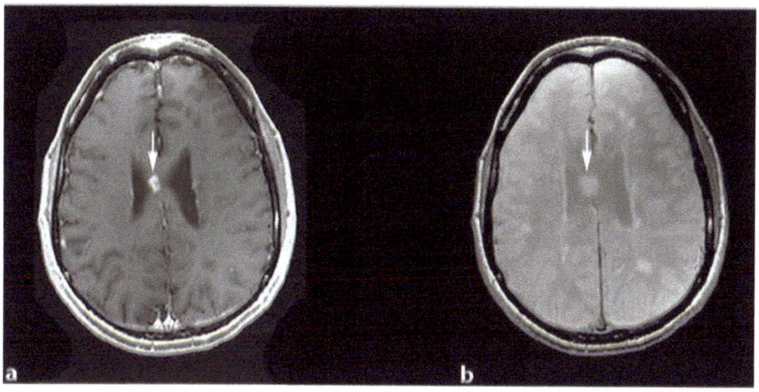

Fig. 3.28 Axial T1-weighted with contrast (**a**) and PD (**b**) images of a patient with RRMS demonstrate an enhancing lesion in the body of corpus callosum (*arrows*)

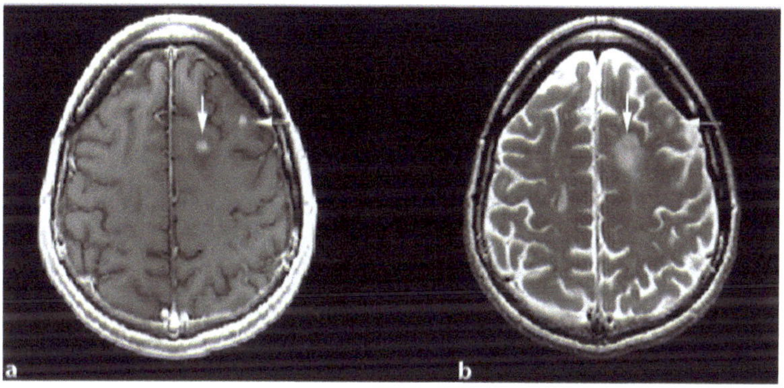

Fig. 3.29 Axial T1-weighted with contrast (**a**) and T2-weighted (**b**) images of a patient with RRMS demonstrate two nodular enhancing lesions with corresponding T2 hyperintensities, one in the deep white matter (*arrows* ↓) and the other in the cortical area (*arrows* ←). Note: Cortical lesions usually do not produce severe edema, but acute lesions in the deep white matter may show a significant amount of edema

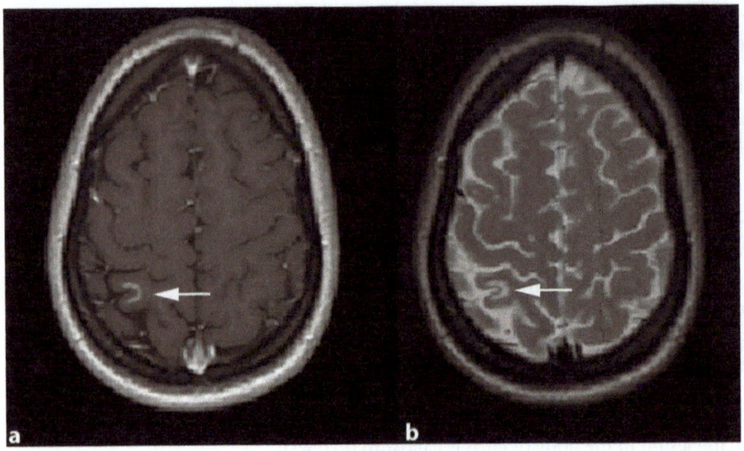

Fig. 3.30 Axial T1-weighted with Gd (**a**) and the corresponding T2-weighted (**b**) images demonstrating enhancement including the U-fibers (*arrows*)

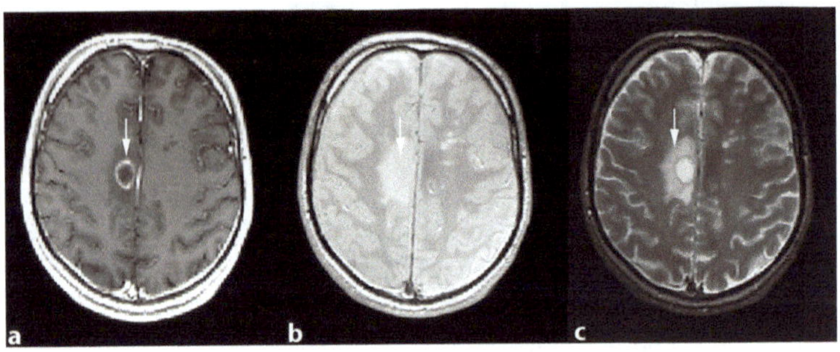

Fig. 3.31 Axial T1-weighted with Gd (**a**), PD- (**b**), and T2-weighted (**c**) images of a patient with MS demonstrate a complete ring enhancing lesion involving the right precentral/frontal cortex and the juxtacortical area (*arrows*)

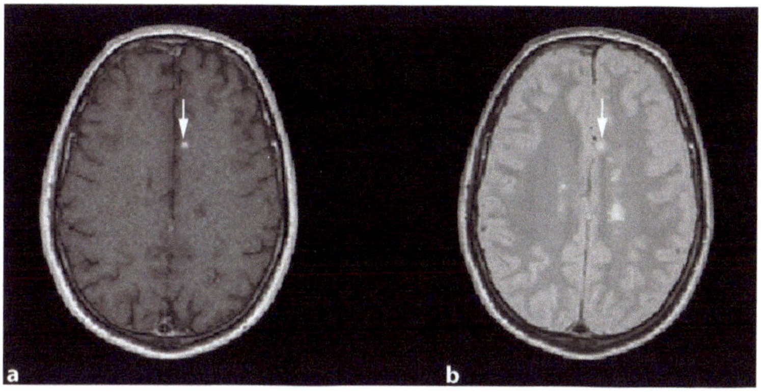

Fig. 3.32 Axial T1-weighted (**a**) and the corresponding T2-weighted (**b**) images demonstrate a cortical enhancing lesion. Note: It is likely that PD- and T2-weighted images miss cortical lesions because of relatively high signal from cortex and partial volume effects, but Gd enhancement can detect acute suspected cortical lesions

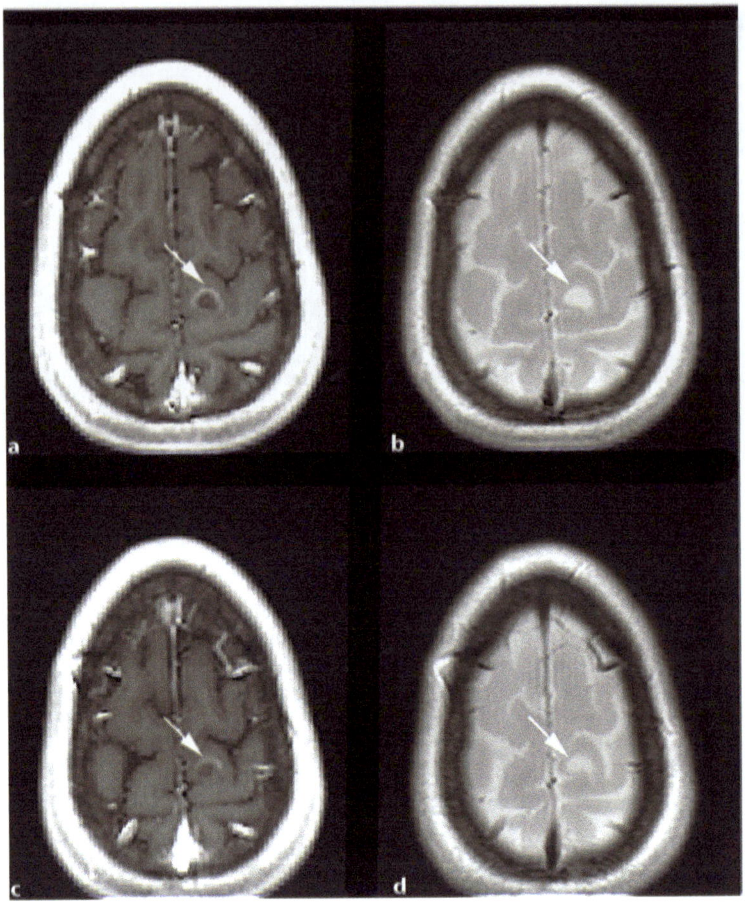

Fig. 3.33 Axial T1-weighted with contrast (**a**,**c**) and corresponding PD (**b**,**d**) images of a patient with MS demonstrate an ring-enhancing lesion in the vertex. Note: a MRI of a patient with MS should cover the whole brain; otherwise, some lesions especially cortical ones may be missed. An examination with 46 slices (slice thickness 3 mm) without any gap is preferred for baseline and follow-up studies in MS

3.5 Follow-Up

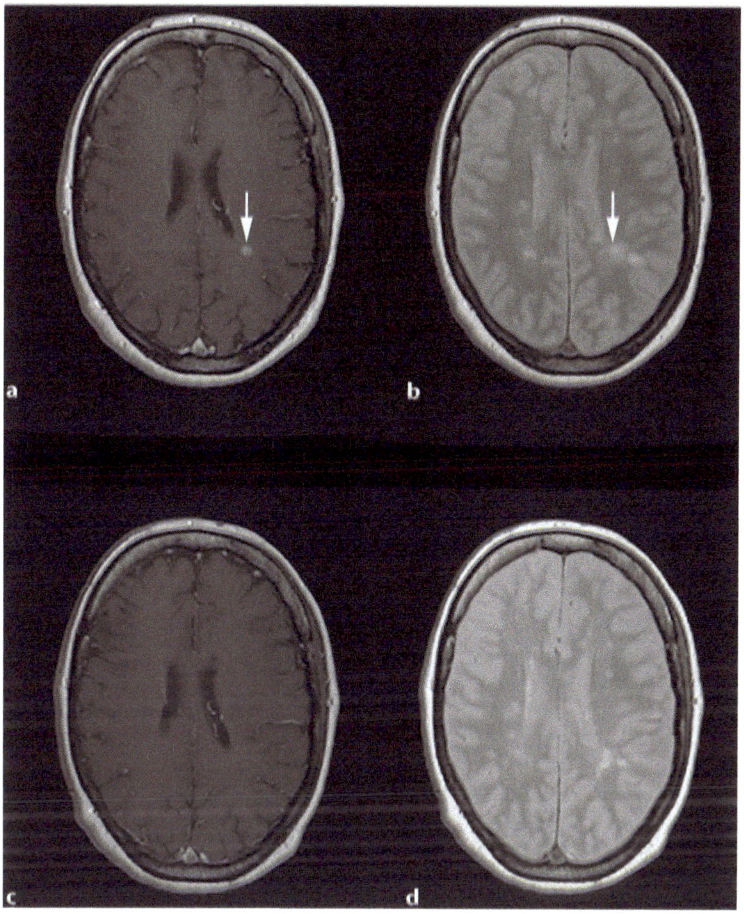

Fig. 3.34 Axial T1-weighted with contrast (**a**) and PD (**b**) images of a patient with RRMS demonstrate a nodular enhancing lesion in the deep white matter of the left parietal lobe (*arrows*). Follow-up images after 1 month (**c**,**d**) demonstrate that the lesion does not show enhancement anymore. Note: In natural history studies most acute lesions lose their enhancement in 4–6 weeks

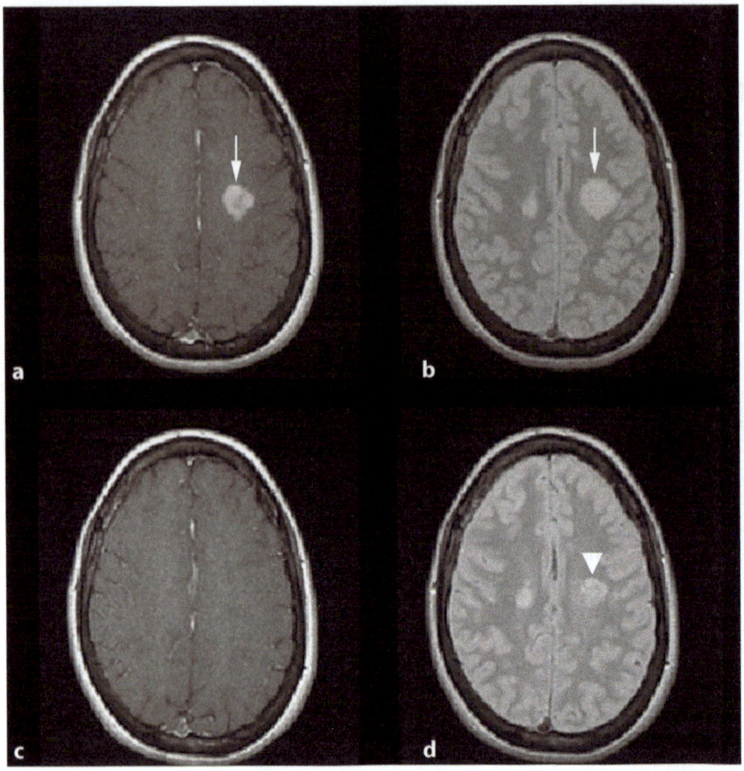

Fig. 3.35 Axial T1-weighted with contrast (**a**) and corresponding PD (**b**) images demonstrate a large enhancing lesion in the deep white matter (*arrows*). Follow-up images after 3 months (**c**,**d**) demonstrate disappearance of the enhancing lesion and a reduction in the size of the PD lesion (*arrowhead*). Note: On contrast-enhanced MR images, MS lesions usually appear as homogeneous oval areas; rarely, however, demyelinating diseases show large contrast enhancing lesions that can be mistaken for tumors. Follow-up images and relative lack of edema help in differentiation

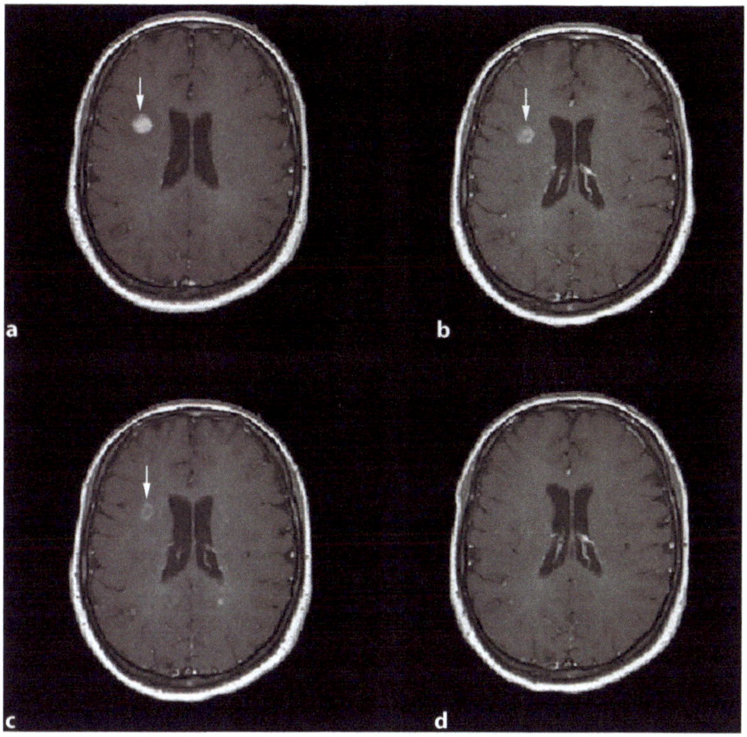

Fig. 3.36 Axial T1-weighted image with contrast demonstrates an enhancing lesion (**a**) and its monthly follow-up (**b–d**). Note: Most enhancing lesions disappear within 4–6 weeks, and it is completely unusual that an enhancing lesion persists for more than 3–4 months

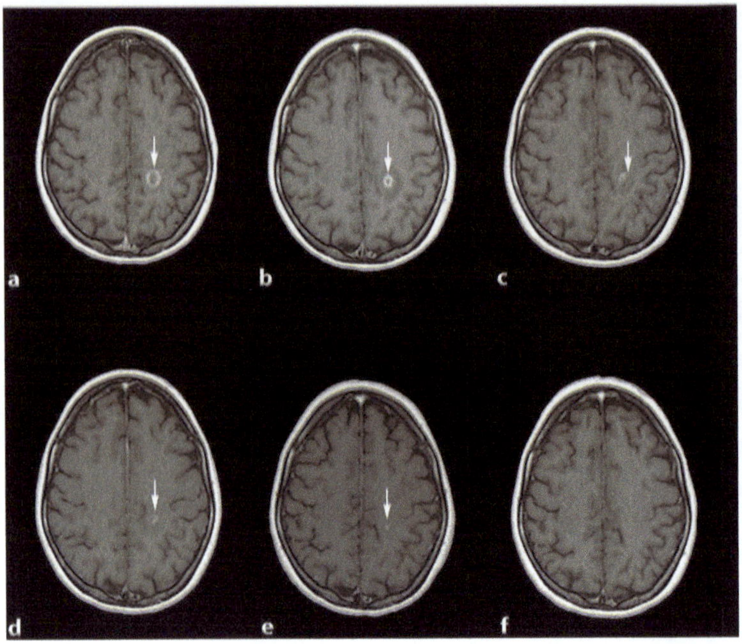

Fig. 3.37 Axial T1-weighted with Gd image of a patient with RRMS demonstrates a ring-enhancing lesion in the deep white matter of the left parietal lobe (**a**) and its monthly follow-up (for 5 months) (**b–f**). The lesion is still present after 4 months (*arrows*) and fades in month 6. Note: As we noted in Fig. 3.36, it is unusual for MS plaques to have Gd enhancement beyond 3 months, although enhancing lesions persisting for 6 months have been rarely reported

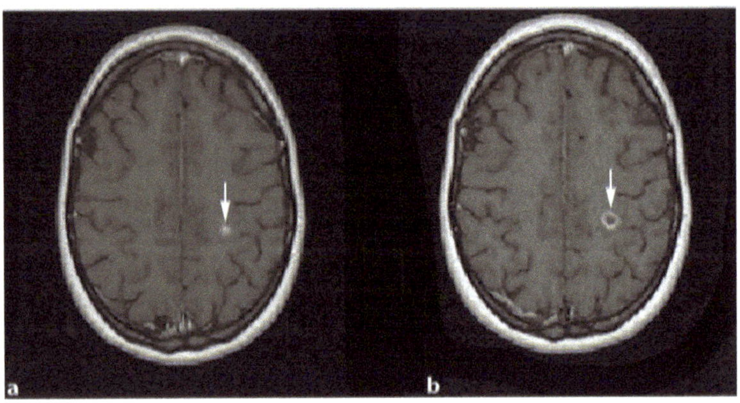

Fig. 3.38 Axial T1-weighted images with Gd (**a**) and its follow-up after 1 month (**b**) demonstrate a nodular enhancing lesion that changed into a ring-enhancing pattern (*arrows*). Note: In longitudinal natural history studies of Gd enhancing lesions, some of the lesions with nodular pattern of enhancement may change into ring enhancing pattern. In fact, potentially more aggressive lesions may change their pattern over one or several weeks

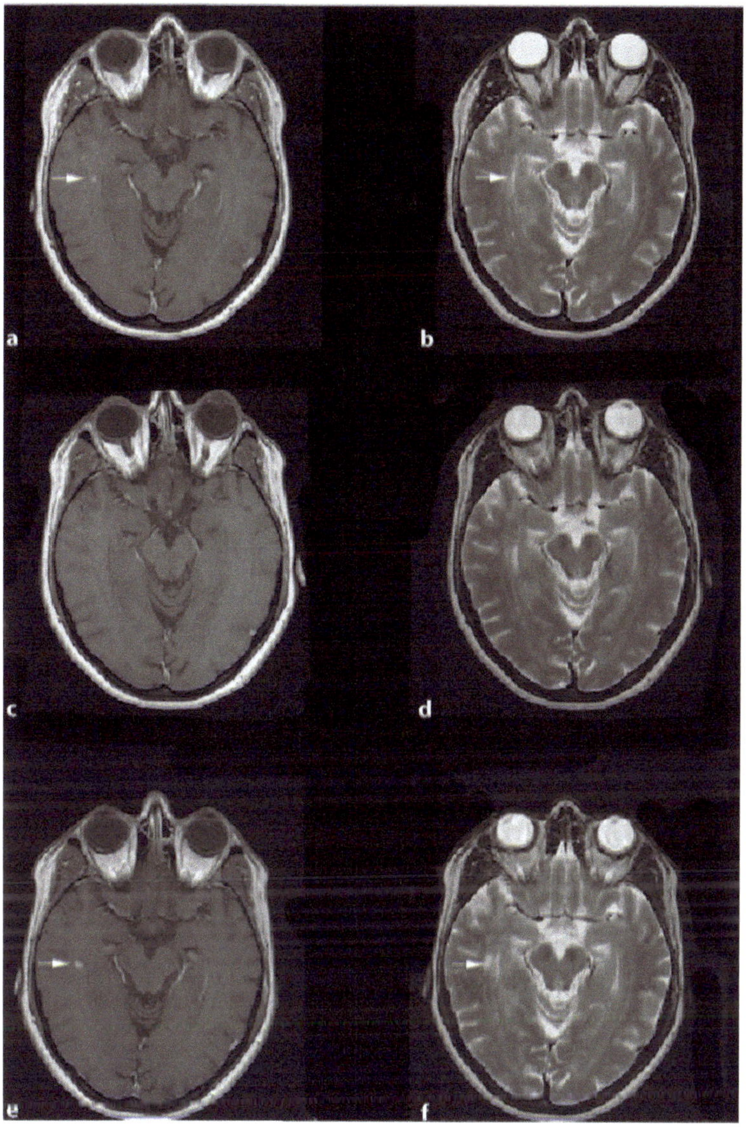

Fig. 3.39 Axial T1-weighted with contrast and T2-weighted images of a patient with RRMS at baseline (**a**,**b**), after 1 month (**c**,**d**), and after 6 months (**e**,**f**) demonstrate re-enhancement of the lesion seen in the baseline after 6 months. The corresponding T2-weighted lesion has also been enlarged. Note: Re-enhancement of old lesions have been seen in less than 5% of MS lesions in longitudinal studies; re-enhancement may be with enlargement in T2-weighted abnormality or not

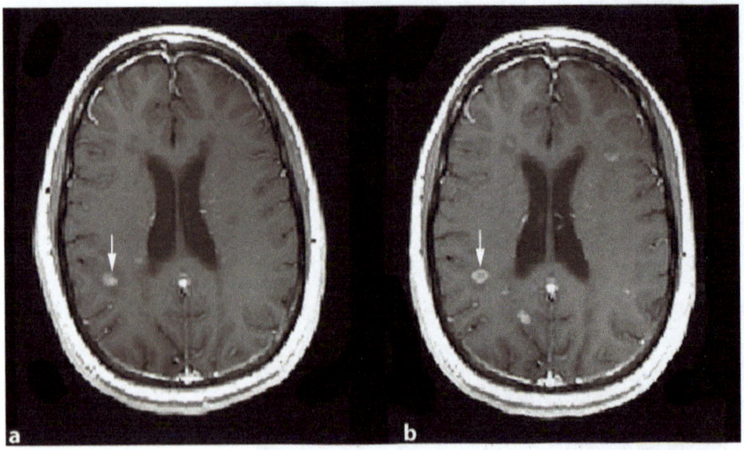

Fig. 3.40 Axial T1-weighted with contrast at baseline (**a**) and after 1 year (**b**) demonstrate two new enhancing lesions and re-enhancement of a previously active lesion (*arrows*)

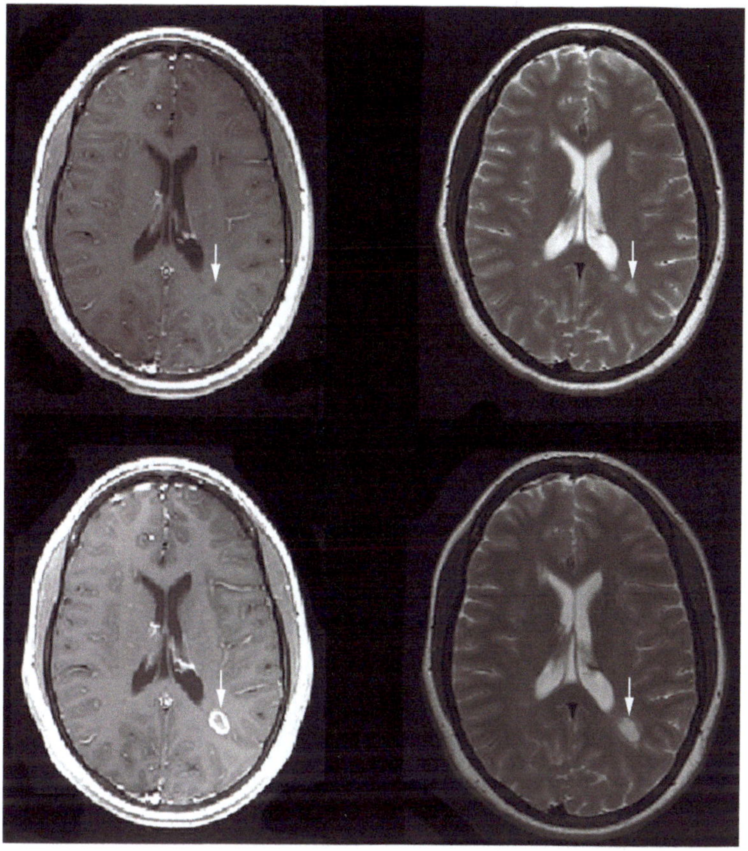

Fig. 3.41 Axial T1-weighted with contrast and PD images of a patient with RRMS at baseline (*upper images*) and after 1 year (*lower images*) demonstrate re-enhancement of a previously old inactive lesion, which is indicative of new inflammatory activity (*arrows*). Note the enlargement of the T2 corresponding lesion after enhancement

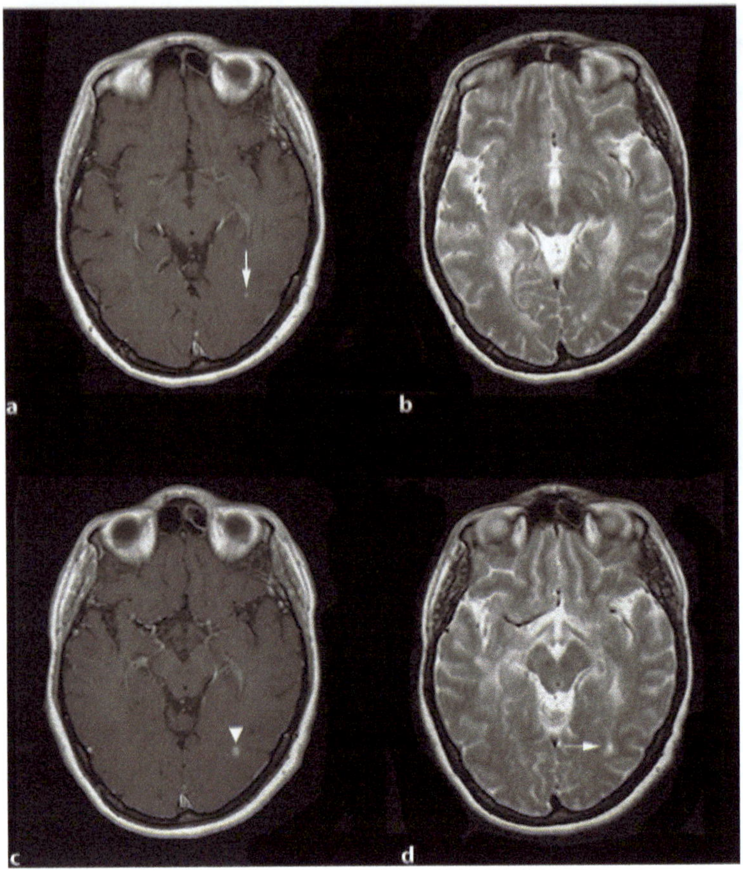

Fig. 3.42 Axial T1-weighted with contrast (**a**) and corresponding T2-weighted (**b**) images of a patient with RRMS demonstrate a tiny enhancing lesion (*arrow*). Follow-up images after 1 month (**c,d**) demonstrate that the size of the lesion has increased (*arrowhead*)

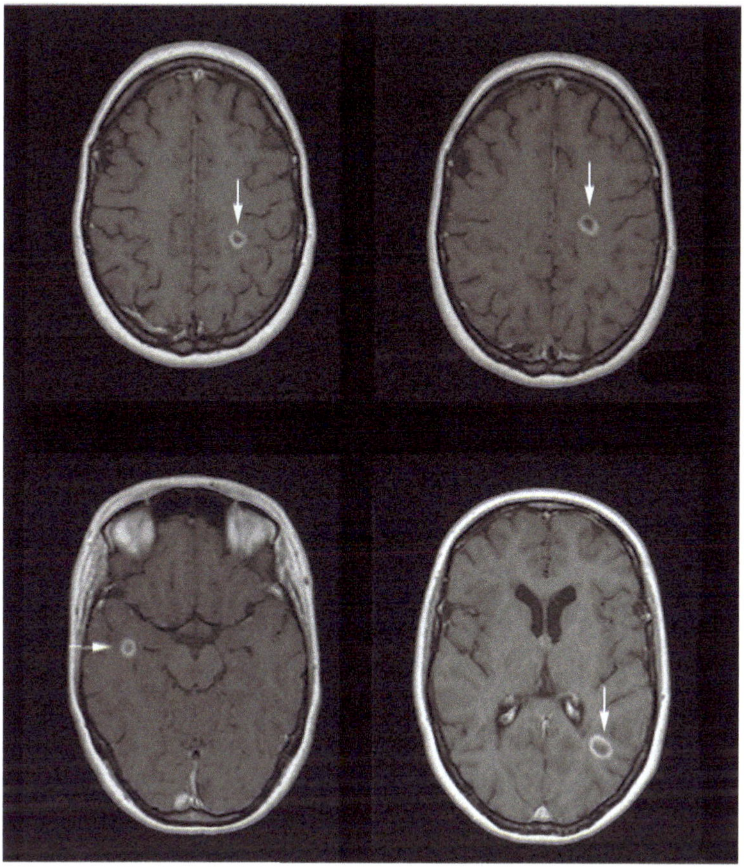

Fig. 3.43 Axial T1-weighted images with Gd in a patient with RRMS demonstrate several ring enhancing lesions in different regions in the follow-up. Note: Ring enhancing lesions seem to be more destructive and may cause severe axonal loss. Some genetic background may be responsible

References

1. Bastianello S, Pozzilli C, Bernardi S et al (1990) Serial study of gadolinium-DTPA MRI enhancement in multiple sclerosis. Neurology 40:591–595
2. Bitsch A, Bruck W (2002) MRI-pathological correlates in MS. Int MSJ 8:89–95
3. Filippi M, Rovaris M, Rocca MA et al (2001) European/Canadian Glatiramer Acetate Study Group. Glatiramer acetate reduces the proportion of new MS lesions evolving into "black holes." Neurology 57:731–733
4. He J, Grossman RI, Ge Y et al (2001) Enhancing patterns in multiple sclerosis: evolution and persistence. AJNR Am J Neuroradiol 22:664–669
5. Kappos L (1999) Multiple sclerosis trials. Lancet 353:2242–2243
6. Kappos L, Moeri D, Radue EW, Schoetzau A, Jordan P, MAGNIMS (1999) Predictive value of gadolinium-enhanced MRI for relapse rate and in development of disability in multiple sclerosis – a metaanalysis. Lancet 353:964–969
7. Miller DH, Grossman RI, Reingold SC (1998) The role of magnetic resonance techniques in understanding and managing multiple sclerosis. Brain 121:3–24
8. Polman C, Reingold SC, Edan G et al (2005) Diagnostic criteria for multiple sclerosis: 2005 revisions to the McDonald Criteria. Ann Neurol 58:840–846
9. Waesberghe JH van, van Walderveen MA, Castelijns JA et al (1998) Patterns of lesion development in multiple sclerosis: longitudinal observations with T1-weighted spin-echo and magnetization transfer MR. AJNR Am J Neuroradiol 19:675–683

4 T1 Hypointense Lesions (Black Holes)

M.A. Sahraian, E.-W. Radue

4.1 Introduction

A black hole (BH) is defined as any abnormal hypointensity as compared with normal-appearing white matter visible on T1-weighted sequences concordant with a region of high signal intensity on T2-weighted images. Black holes are considered to be acute when they coincide with a contrast enhancing lesion (CEL), and to be chronic or persistent when no corresponding CEL exists (Bagnato et al. 2003).

Some authors consider *true chronic black holes* as hypointense lesions, which do not show contrast enhancement and persist for more than 6 months. Here we consider chronic black holes as hypointense lesions that do not enhance after contrast injection on T1-weighted images.

T1 hypointense lesions were first described by Ulhenbrock et al. (1989), who noted that they were more common in MS than in subcortical arteriosclerotic encephalopathy. T1 black holes typically show enhancement in the beginning and evolve differently from patient to patient and even within the same patient. Their signal intensities vary from deep gray – like cerebrospinal fluid to light gray – like cerebral cortex. Approximately 65–80% of CELs appear hypointense on unenhanced T1-weighted images (van Waesberghe et al. 1998; Bakshi et al. 2005) and when contrast enhancement disappears, these black holes may become isointense to the normal-appearing white matter or develop hypointensities (14–41%). The longevity of persistent BHs may vary after contrast enhancement. Some lesions may be visible for a relatively short period of time, some enlarge or shrink, and some others may eventually maintain hypointensity (Bagnato et al. 2003). Contrast enhancing lesions persisting for more than 1 month and ring enhancing lesions have a greater chance to evolve into chronic black holes.

T1 hypointensity is in principle caused by an expansion of the extracellular space due to an increase in water content and a loss of structural components. Pathologically, this may be a consequence of tissue destruction or of an increase in water influx. In fact, the pathological correlations of T1 hypointense lesions depend, in part, on the lesion age. Newly formed hypointense lesions likely reflect variable combination of inflammation, edema, demyelination, early remyelination, axonal transection, and glial activation. Lesions that show most profound hypointensity on T1-weighted images correlate pathologically with the most profound demyelination and axonal loss (Bitsch and Bruck 2002).

There are several different reports about the correlation of T1-weighted black holes and clinical disability. In some studies, T1 lesion load showed a higher correlation with the expanded disability status scale (EDSS) for patients with RRMS than in patients with the secondary progressive type in cross-sectional studies (Goodin 2006).

Looking at the T1/T2 lesion load, several studies have demonstrated a lower ratio in patients with RRMS compared with the secondary progressive type of the disease (van Walderveen et al. 1999).

Longitudinal changes of T1 hypointense lesion volume have been investigated in some clinical trials during recent years to see if the drugs can prevent axonal loss irrespective of a decrease in enhancing lesions.

In this chapter we demonstrate different types of black holes of different sizes and intensities and in various anatomical sites. We show the evolution of persisting lesions by demonstrating serial imaging of patients.

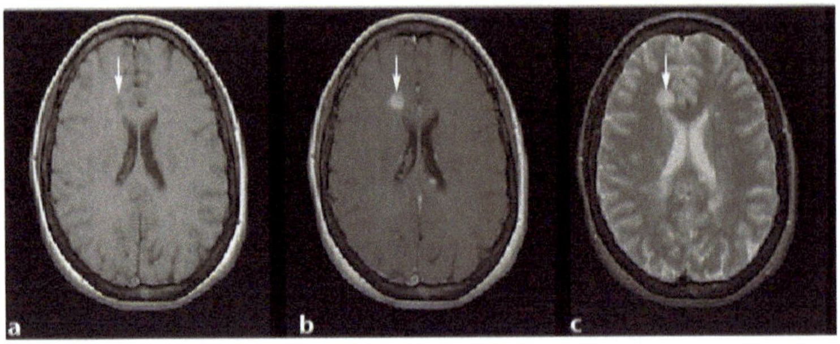

Fig. 4.1 Axial T1-weighted without (**a**), with contrast (**b**), and corresponding T2-weighted (**c**) images of a patient with RRMS demonstrate a hypointense lesion on T1 without contrast that has been enhanced after Gd injection. Note: Acute black holes are defined as hypointense lesions on native T1-weighted images when they correspond to enhancing lesions on T1-weighted with contrast

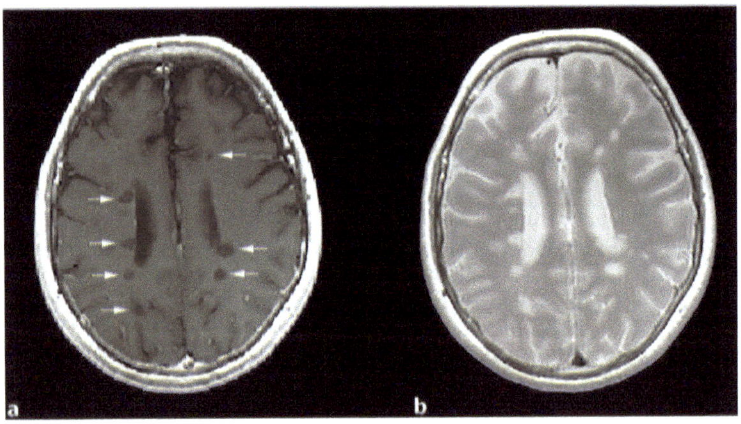

Fig. 4.2 Axial T1-weighted with contrast (**a**) and corresponding PD (**b**) images of a patient with RRMS demonstrate several hypointense lesions on the T1-weighted image (*arrows*). Note: Only a subset of T2 hyperintense lesions may appear hypointense on T1-weighted images. All of these hypointense lesions have corresponding T2-weighted abnormalities

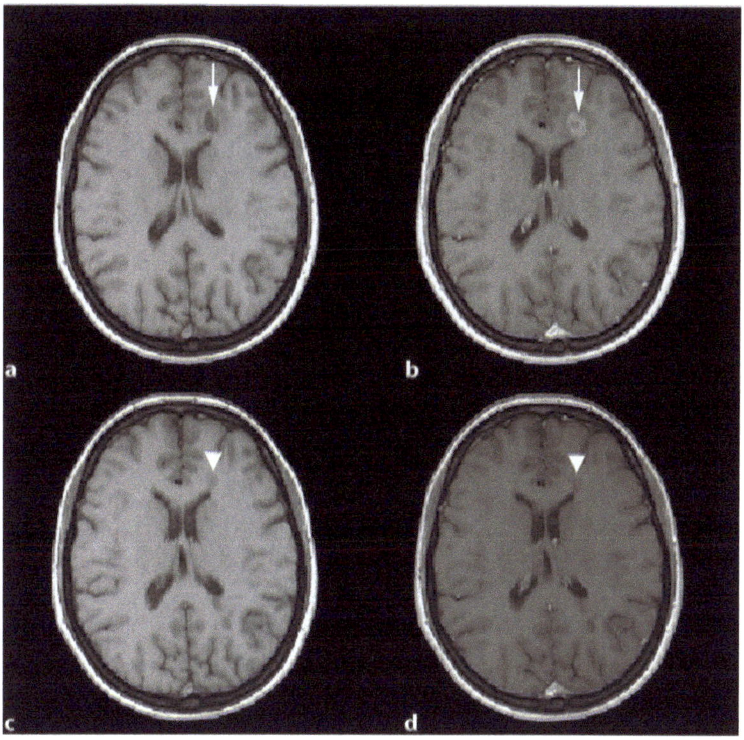

Fig. 4.3 Axial T1-weighted without (**a**) and with (**b**) contrast images demonstrate an acute hypointense lesion on the T1-weighted image with the corresponding enhancing lesions (*arrows*). Follow-up images after 6 months (**c,d**) demonstrate that the contrast-enhanced lesion has disappeared, but a hypointense lesion has developed on the T1-weighted image with contrast (*arrowheads*). Note: Hypointense lesions that persist for a minimum of 6 months after their first appearance are called persistent or chronic black holes. These lesions seem to be associated with greater tissue destruction and axonal loss

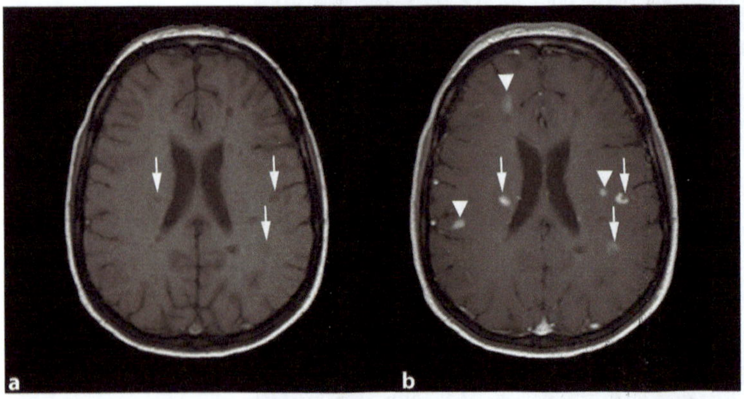

Fig. 4.4 Axial T1-weighted image without (**a**) and with contrast (**b**) images of a patient with RRMS demonstrate several enhancing lesions on the T1-weighted with contrast. Some of these enhancing lesions appear hypointense on T1-weighted without contrast (*arrows*), and some of them appear isointense (*arrowheads*). Note: Approximately 80% of the enhancing lesions appear hypointense on T1-weighted image without contrast

4.2 Shape and Size

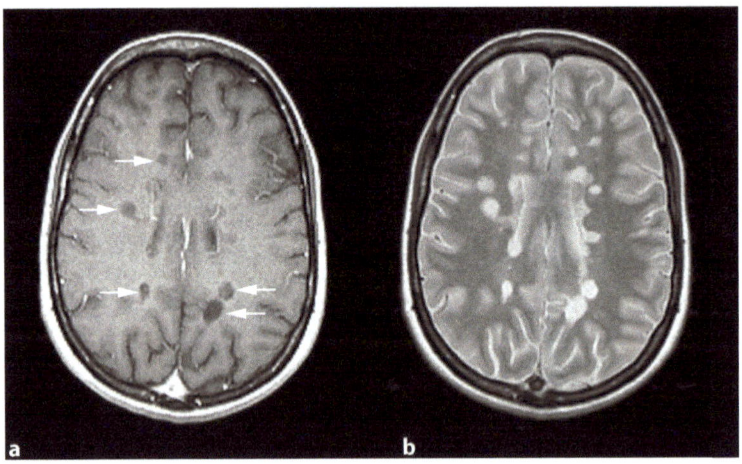

Fig. 4.5 Axial T1-weighted with contrast (**a**) and PD (**b**) images demonstrate several black holes with different signal intensities distributed over the white matter (*arrows*). Note: The range of hypointensity is completely variable; some lesions are nearly like CSF and others are close to gray matter. The degree of hypointensity may have correlation with axonal loss and structural damage

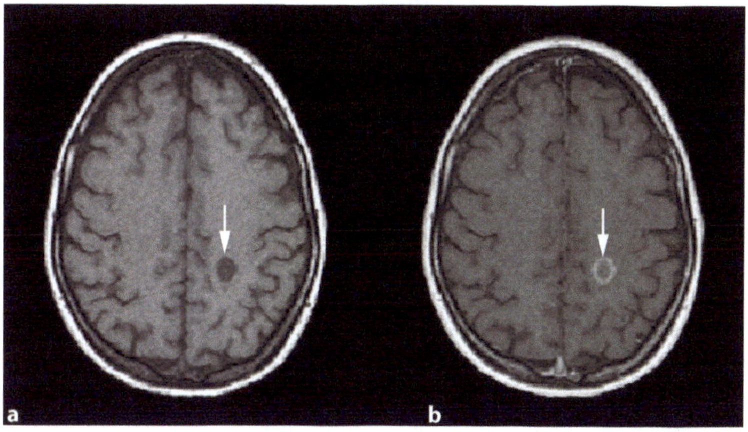

Fig. 4.6 Axial T1-weighted without (**a**) and with contrast-enhanced (**b**) images demonstrate an acute hypointense lesion that shows ring enhancement after contrast injection (*arrows*). Note: Ring enhancing lesions have a higher probability to demonstrate hypointensity on T1-weighted images as compared with other patterns of enhancement

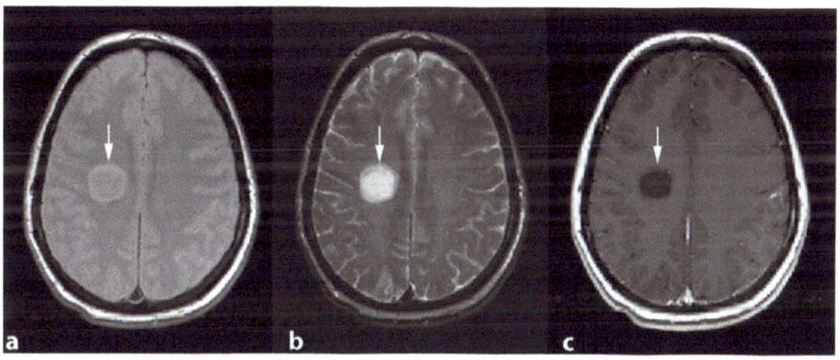

Fig. 4.7 Axial PD (**a**), T2 weighted (**b**), and T1-weighted with contrast (**c**) images demonstrate a large MS lesion that is severely hypointense on the T1-weighted image with contrast (*arrows*). Note: Black holes usually have a small diameter, but some cases may show large or confluent black holes

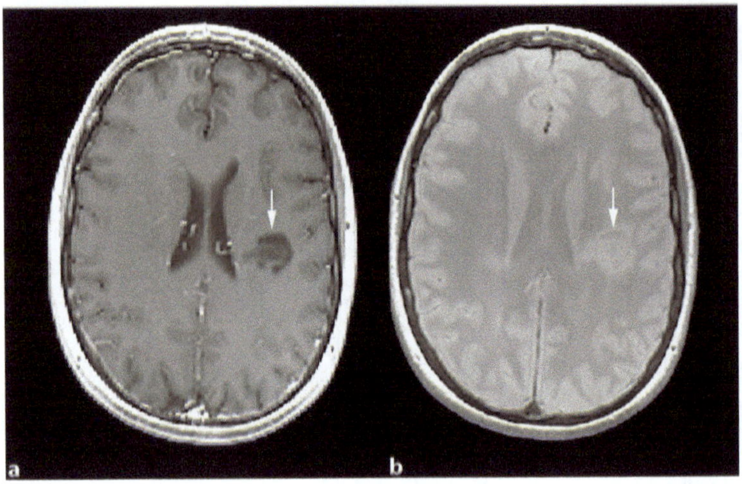

Fig. 4.8 Axial T1-weighted with contrast (**a**) and PD (**b**) images demonstrate a large black hole with different signal intensities (*arrows*)

4.3 Locations

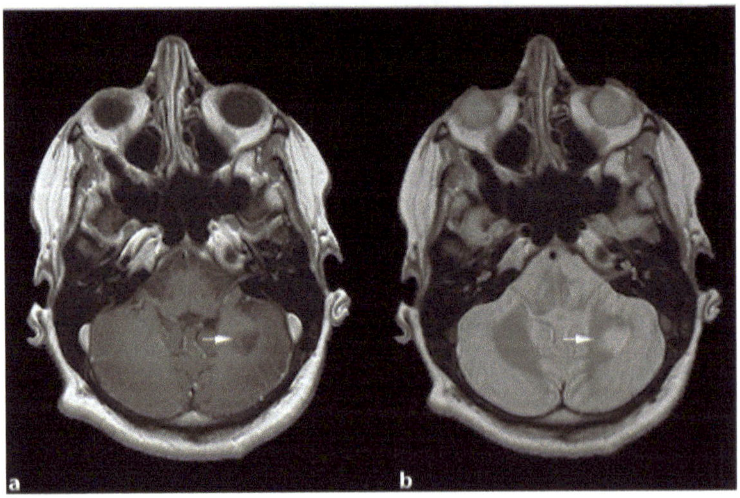

Fig. 4.9 Axial T1-weighted with contrast (**a**) and PD (**b**) images demonstrate a large black hole in the left cerebellar hemisphere, with corresponding T2-hyperintensity (*arrows*)

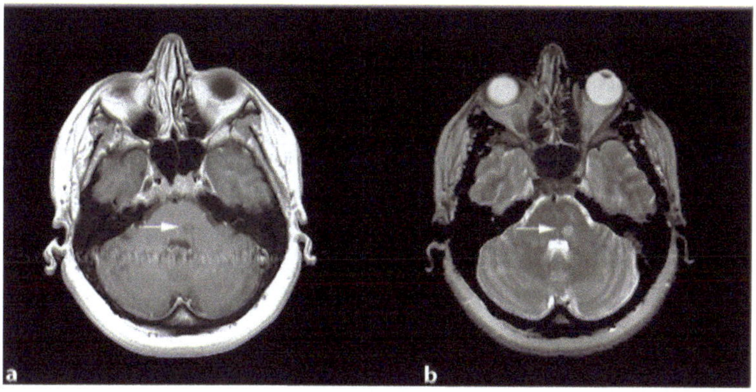

Fig. 4.10 Axial T1-weighted with Gd (**a**) and corresponding T2-weighted (**b**) images demonstrate a chronic black hole of the pons and its T2 hyperintensity (*arrows*)

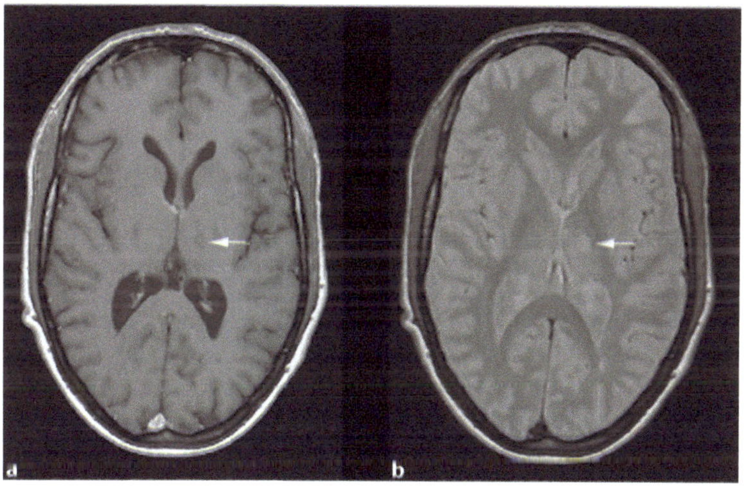

Fig. 4.11 Axial T1-weighted with contrast (**a**) and PD (**b**) images demonstrate a black hole in the thalamus. The corresponding hyperintense lesion can be seen on the PD image (*arrows*)

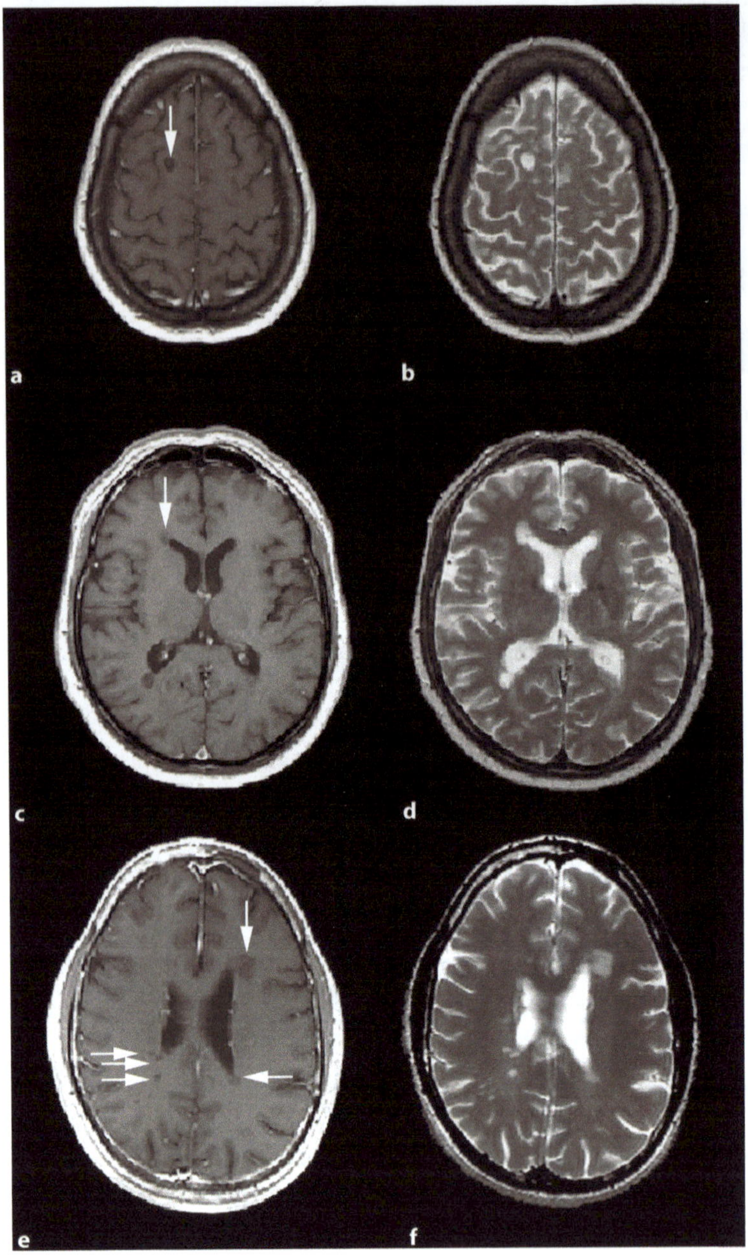

Fig. 4.12 Axial T1-weighted with contrast (**a**,**c**,**e**) and T2-weighted (**b**,**d**,**f**) images demonstrate several black holes with different signal intensities, sizes, and in various locations

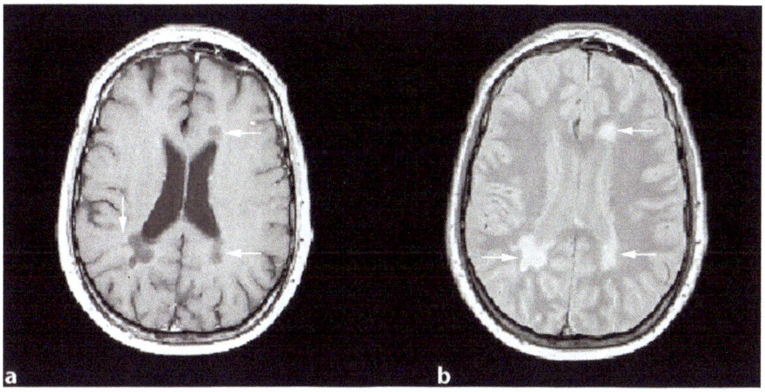

Fig. 4.13 Axial T1-weighted (**a**) and PD (**b**) images demonstrate periventricular black holes with the corresponding T2 abnormalities (*arrows*)

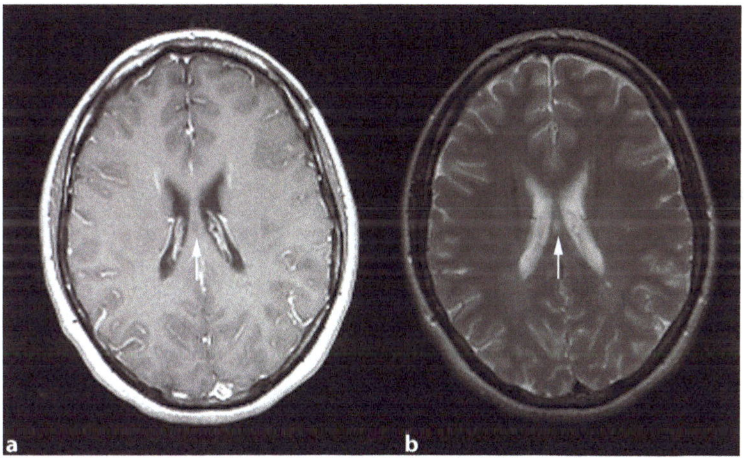

Fig. 4.14 Axial T1-weighted with contrast (**a**) and T2-weighted (**b**) images demonstrate a black hole of the corpus callosum (*arrows*)

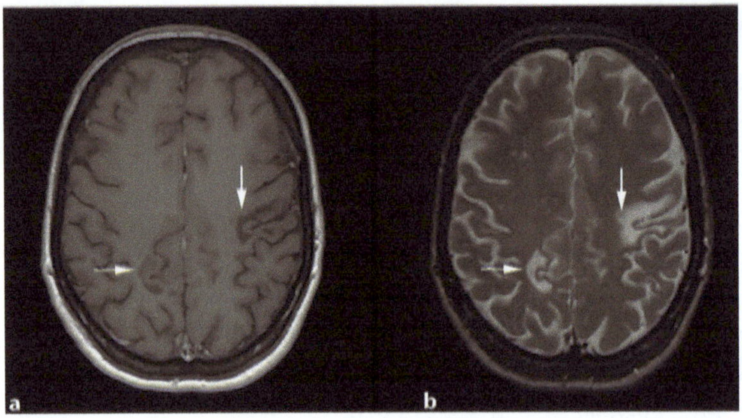

Fig. 4.15 Axial T1-weighted with contrast (**a**) and T2-weighted (**b**) images demonstrate two juxtacortical black holes involving U-fibers with corresponding T2-weighted abnormalities (*arrows*)

4.4 Follow-Up

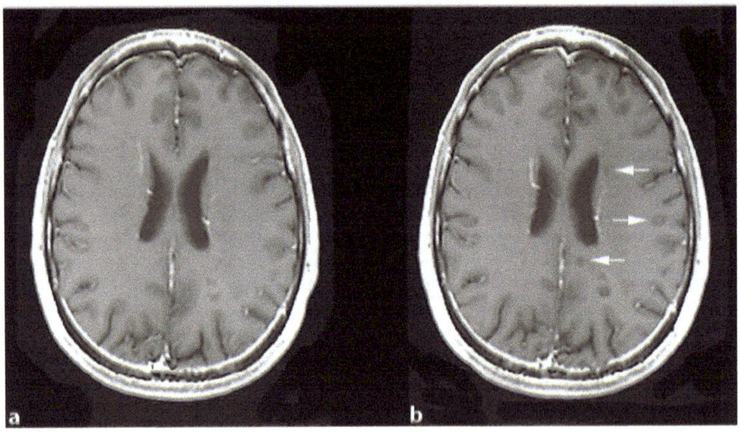

Fig. 4.16 Axial T1-weighted with contrast images at baseline (**a**) and follow-up after 1 year (**b**) demonstrate new black holes (*arrows*). Note: It is not clear why some enhancing lesions may result in black holes and others change into isointensity. It should also be noted that some patients may develop more black holes than do others. Genetic susceptibility has been proposed as one of the factors

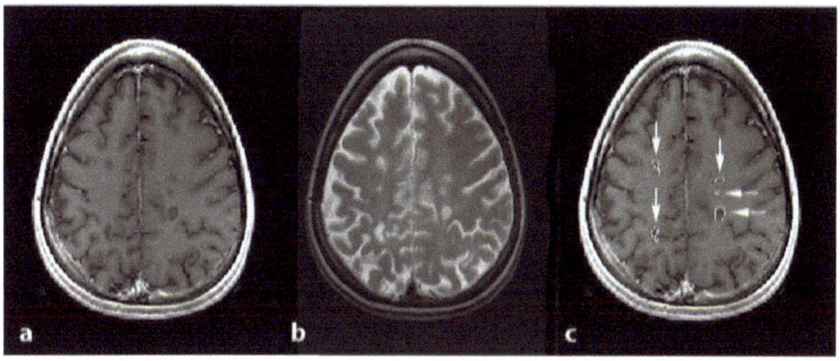

Fig. 4.17 Axial T1-weighted with contrast (**a**) and PD (**b**) images of a patient with MS demonstrate black holes segmentation (**c**) (*arrows*). Note: Changes in the volume of black holes have been recently used as a surrogate marker in some clinical trials to show the potency of drugs in preventing structural damage and axonal loss

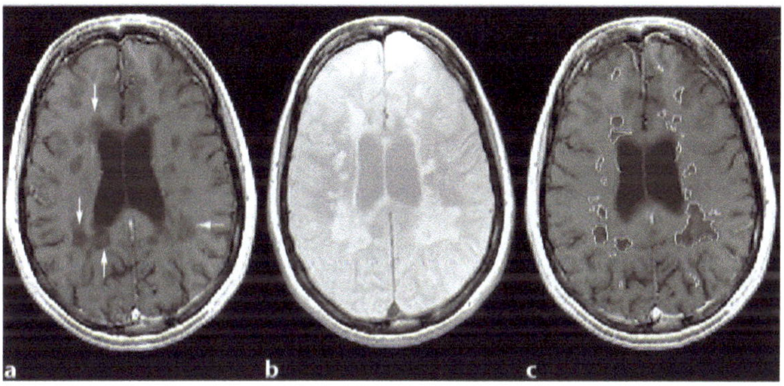

Fig. 4.18 Axial T1-weighted with contrast (**a**), PD- (**b**), and T1-weighted (**c**) images of a patient with Secondary Progressive MS (SPMS) demonstrate several black holes with corresponding PD abnormalities. Segmentation of the black holes is demonstrated in **c**. This patient has a large volume of black holes. Note: The T1/T2 lesion ratio is higher in secondary progressive MS than in RRMS

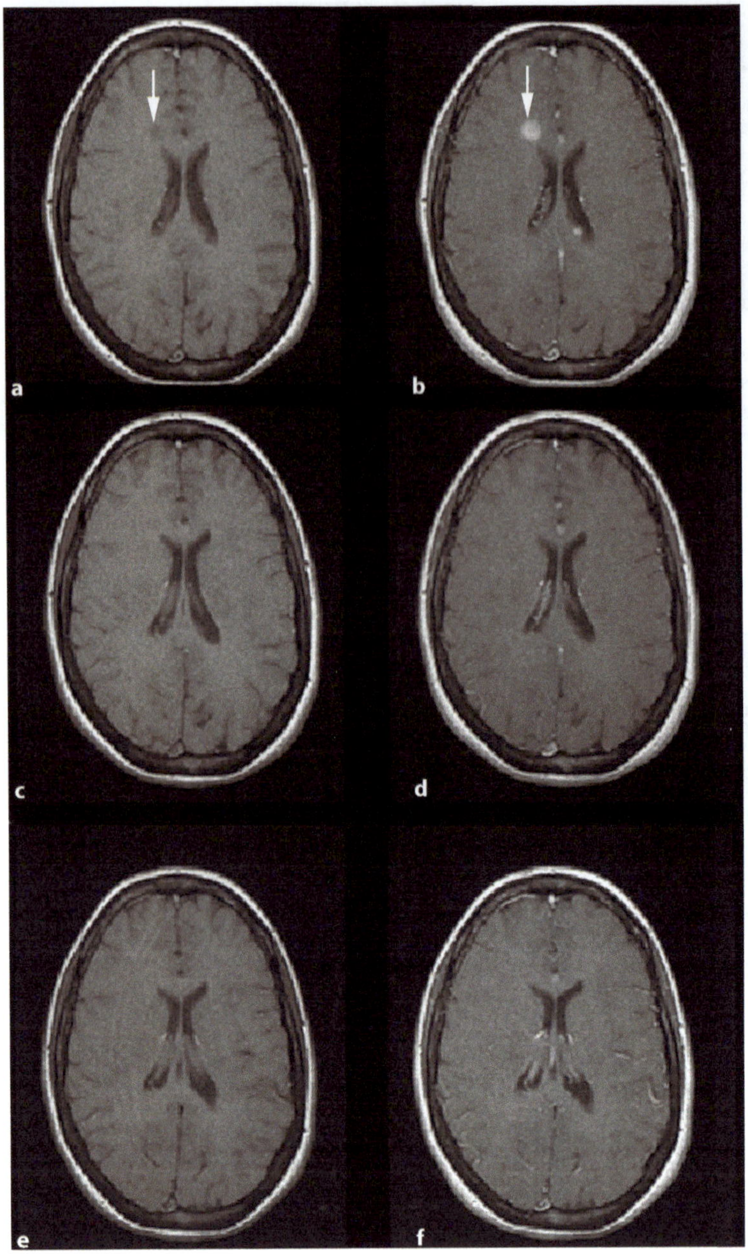

Fig. 4.19 Axial T1-weighted images without (**a**) and with contrast (**b**) demonstrate an acute black hole and the corresponding enhancing lesion (*arrows*). Follow-up images after 1 (**c**,**d**) and 6 months (**e**,**f**) demonstrate that the acute hypointensity and the enhancing lesions have disappeared. Note: Most acute black holes increase their intensity and become isointense within 6 months, and less than 40% become persistent hypointensities

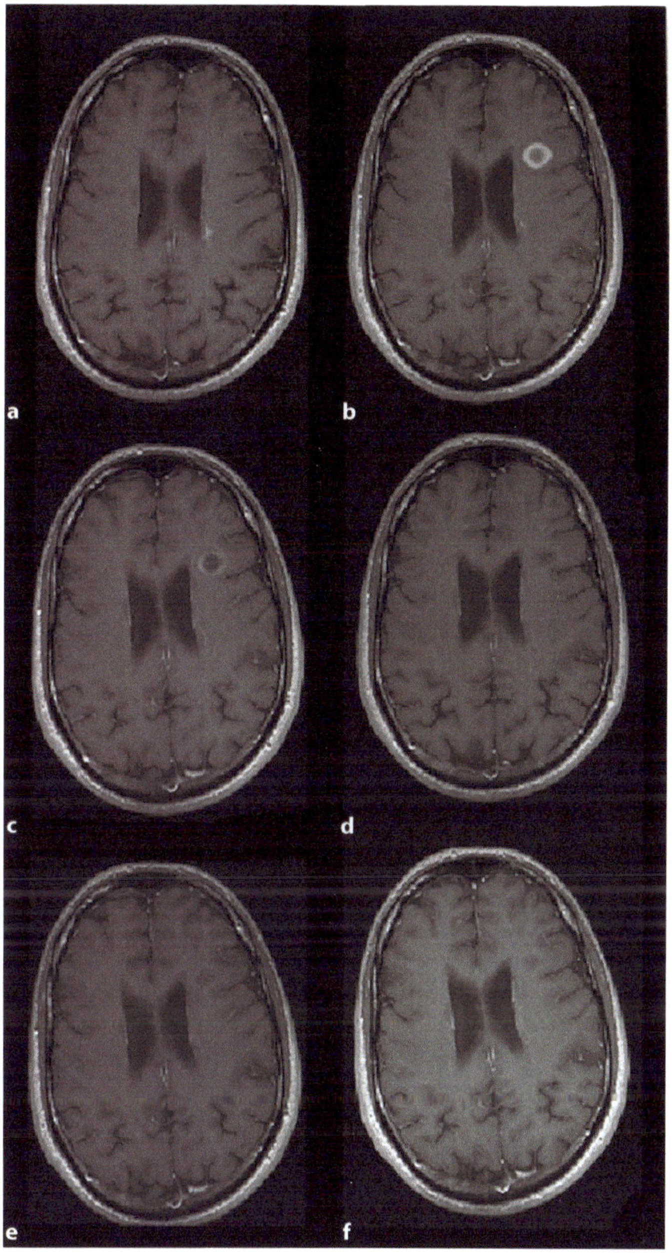

Fig. 4.20 Axial T1-weighted with contrast images demonstrate baseline and follow-up images of a patient with RRMS. On the baseline image (**a**) there is no Gd enhancing lesion, in month 1 the patient developed a ring enhancing lesion (**b**) that was persistent in month 2 (**c**) and changed into a hypointense lesion without enhancement in month 3 (**d**). Follow-up images after 6 months (**e**) and 1 year (**f**) show that the black hole is still present although signal intensity increased slightly

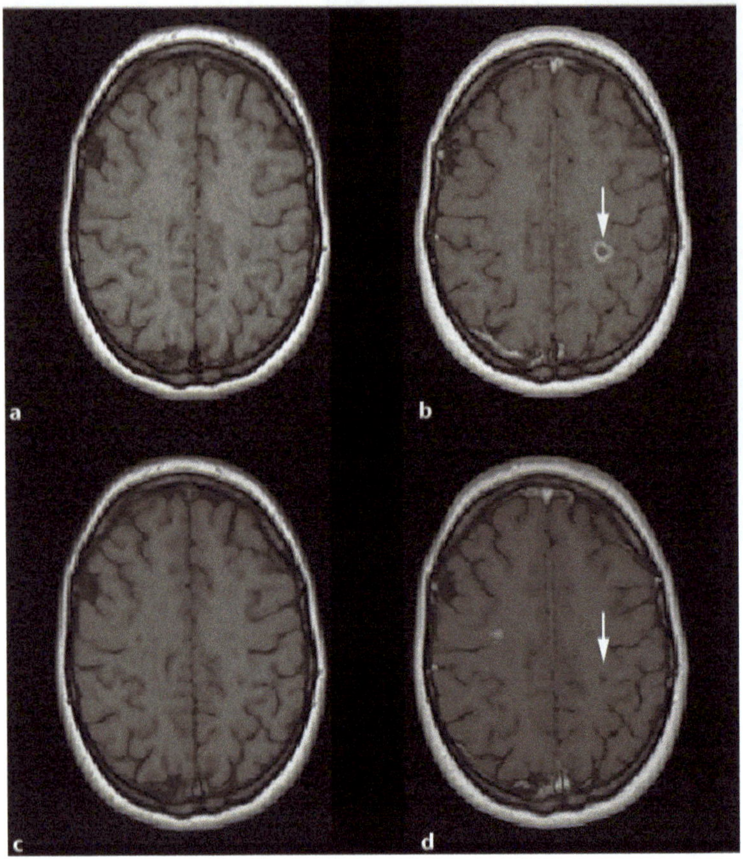

Fig. 4.21 Axial T1-weighted without (**a,c**) and with contrast (**b,d**) images of a patient with MS demonstrate an acute black hole with corresponding ring enhancing lesion. After 6 months the hypointense lesion is still persistent (**c,d**) (*arrows*). Note: Ring enhancing lesions have a higher probability to develop into chronic black holes than other patterns of enhancement

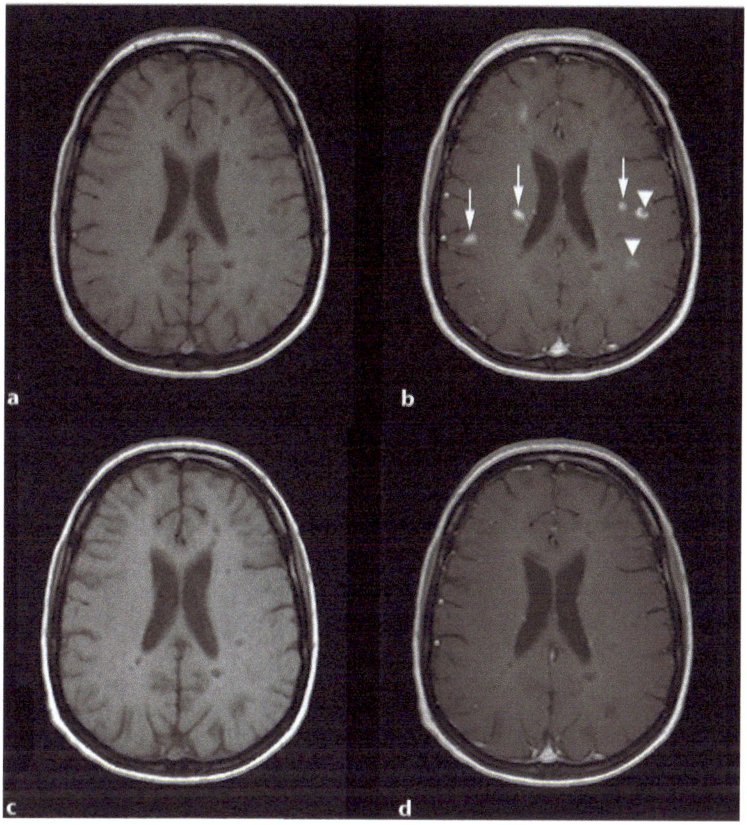

Fig. 4.22 Axial T1-weighted without (**a,c**) and with (**b,d**) contrast images demonstrate baseline (*upper images*) and follow-up (*lower images*) of a patient with RRMS. In the baseline images the patient has several Gd enhancing lesions (four of them have been marked by *arrows*) and some acute black holes. After 6 months, only one of the previously enhanced lesions has kept its signal intensity, i.e., changed into a chronic black hole

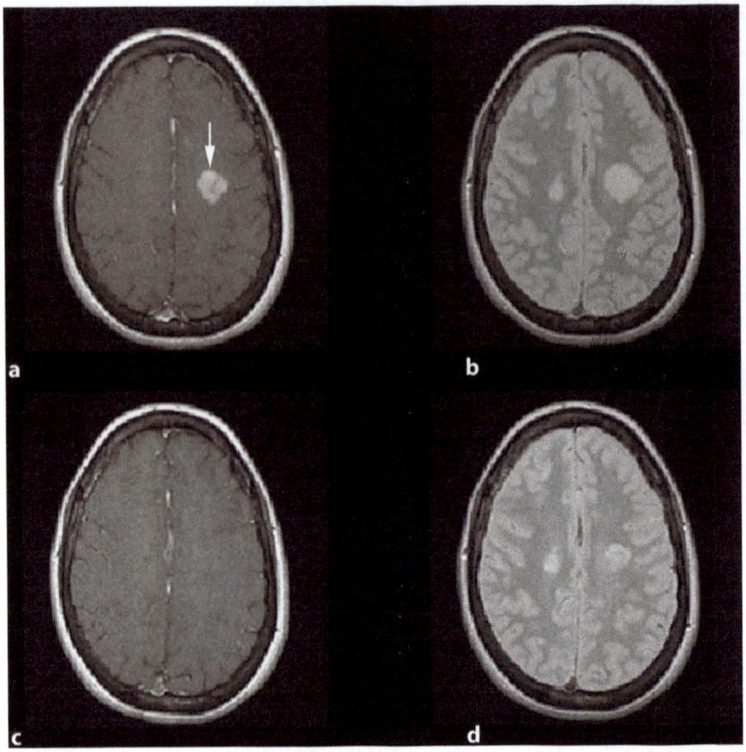

Fig. 4.23 Axial T1-weighted without (**a,c**) and with (**b,d**) contrast images, baseline (*upper images*) and follow-up (*lower images*) of a patient with RRMS demonstrate a large enhancing lesion (*arrow*) that has become isointense after 6 months

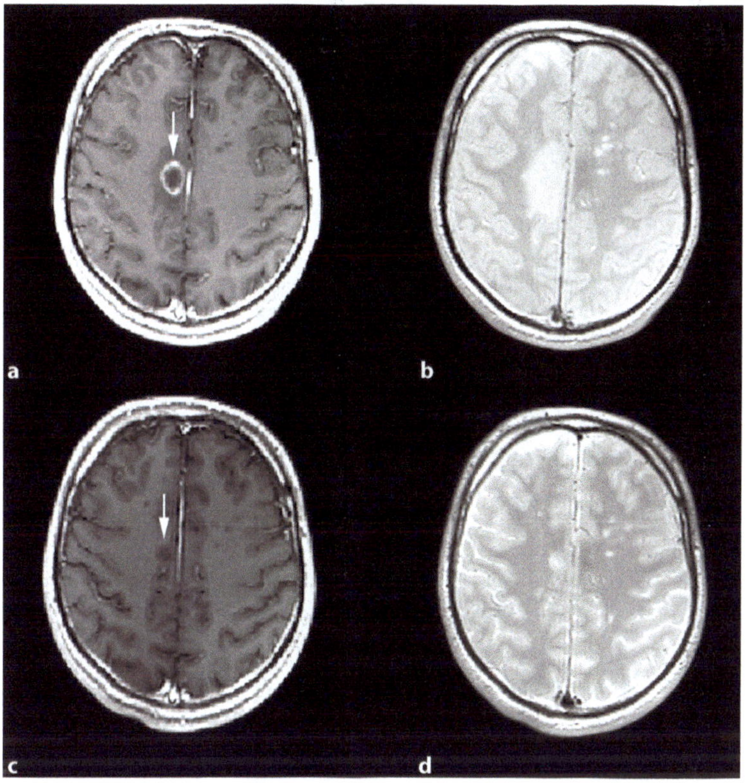

Fig. 4.24 Axial T1-weighted with contrast (**a**,**c**) and PD (**b**,**d**) images, baseline (*upper images*) and follow-up (*lower images*) of a patient with RRMS demonstrate a large cortical ring enhancing lesion (*arrow*) that has become a small cortical black hole after 1 year. Note: Finding cortical black holes is difficult because of similar signal intensity with gray matter and they may be easily missed

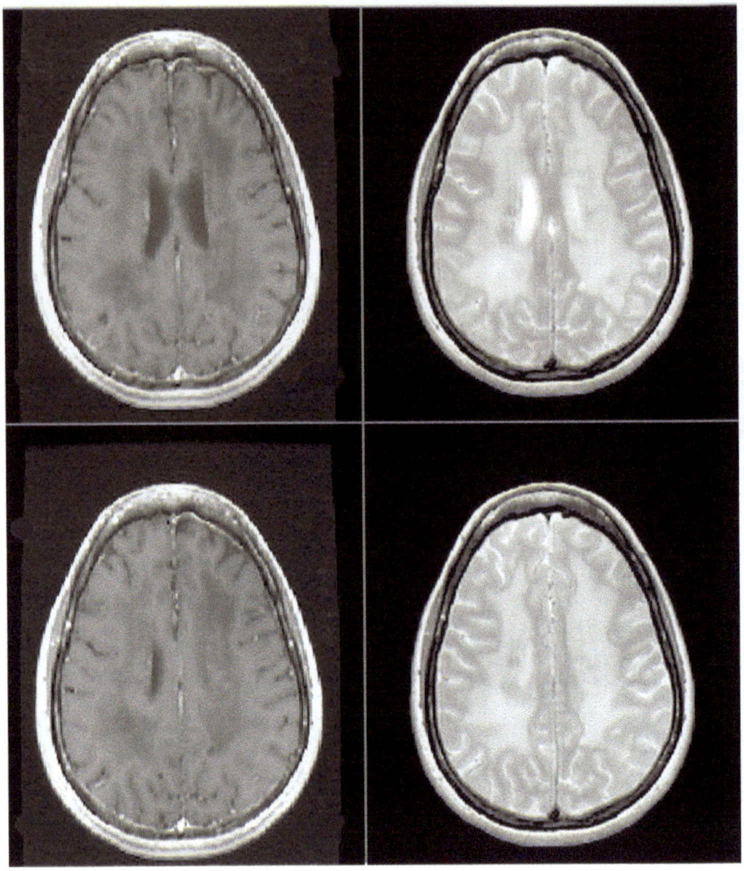

Fig.4.25 Axial T1-weighted with contrast (*left side*) and T2-weighted (*right side*) images demonstrate a large volume of confluent hypointense lesions around the ventricles and deep white matter indicative of extensive tissue destruction

References

1. Bagnato F, Jeffries N, Richert ND et al (2003) Evolution of T1 black holes in patients with multiple sclerosis imaged monthly for 4 years. Brain 126:1782–1789
2. Bakshi R, Minagar A, Jaisani Z et al (2005) Imaging of multiple sclerosis: role in neurotherapeutics. NeuroRx 2:277–303
3. Bitsch A, Bruck W (2002) MRI-pathological correlates in MS. Int MSJ 8:89–95
4. Goodin DS (2006) Magnetic resonance imaging as a surrogate outcome measure of disability in multiple sclerosis: have we been overly harsh in our assessment? Ann Neurol 59:597–605
5. Uhlenbrock D, Sehlen S (1989) The value of T1-weighted images in the differentiation between MS, white matter lesions, and subcortical arteriosclerotic encephalopathy (SAE). Neuroradiology 31:203–212
6. Waesberghe JH van, van Walderveen MA, Castelijns JA et al (1998) Patterns of lesion development in multiple sclerosis: longitudinal observations with T1-weighted spin-echo and magnetization transfer MR. AJNR Am J Neuroradiol 19:675–683
7. Walderveen MA van, Truyen L, van Oosten BW et al (1999) Development of hypointense lesions on T1-weighted spin-echo magnetic resonance images in multiple sclerosis: relation to inflammatory activity. Arch Neurol 56:345–451

5 Multiple Sclerosis and Brain Atrophy

M.A. Sahraian, E.-W. Radue

5.1 Introduction

Atrophy of the brain and spinal cord has been recognized as part of MS pathology for a long time. Several studies have demonstrated annual decrease in brain volume of MS patients, ranging from 0.6 to 1%, compared with 0.1 to 0.3% in the general population during the normal aging process (Comi et al. 2001; Rovaris et al. 2001; Hardmeier et al. 2003; Ge et al. 2000).

The exact mechanism has not been determined, and the etiology seems to be multifactorial. Brain atrophy may result largely from myelin and axonal loss (Ge et al. 2000). Wallerian degeneration, particularly in the neuronal pathways, may also contribute to tissue loss. Atrophy is a progressive phenomenon and seems to be independent of disease subtypes and focal lesion load (Hardmeier et al. 2005; Kalkers et al. 2002). Patients with RRMS tend to lose 17.3 ml a year of brain parenchymal volume (Ge et al. 2000).

The changes that occur over time are relatively small and very sensitive measures are required to detect atrophy, especially on an individual basis. The explanation of these methods is beyond the subject of this chapter, and the reader is referred to the comprehensive reviews on these methods (Miller et al. 2002; Zivadinov et al. 2004).

Application of semiautomated and fully automated image analyses results in more precise measurement of atrophy for longitudinal studies. Different studies suggest that there is only unsignificant correlation between T2 lesion volume, black holes, Gd enhancing lesions and atrophy (Losseff et al. 1996; Paolillo et al. 2000; Zivadinov and Zorzon 2004).

The correlation between brain atrophy and clinical disability seems to be stronger than is T2-lesion load (Dartidar et al. 1999).

Fisher et al. (2002) showed that whole-brain atrophy changes in the first 2 years were the best MRI predictor of the 8-year EDSS score. A number of studies have also established an association between brain atrophy and cognitive impairment in MS patients (Benedict et al. 2004). Furthermore, whole-brain atrophy predicts cognitive impairment in both cross-sectional and longitudinal studies (Benedict et al. 2004; Zivadinov et al. 2001). Atrophy has been considered as a surrogate marker in some clinical trials of MS (Rudic 2004). Although this issue is of growing interest in the therapeutic monitoring of MS, the limitations and challenges (effects of non-disease factors on tissue volume loss) need to be further evaluated. In fact, brain volume changes are complex and may be affected by inflammation, edema, hormonal levels, and medications.

In this chapter, we present several images of patients with MS that demonstrate cerebral atrophy.

5.2 General Atrophy

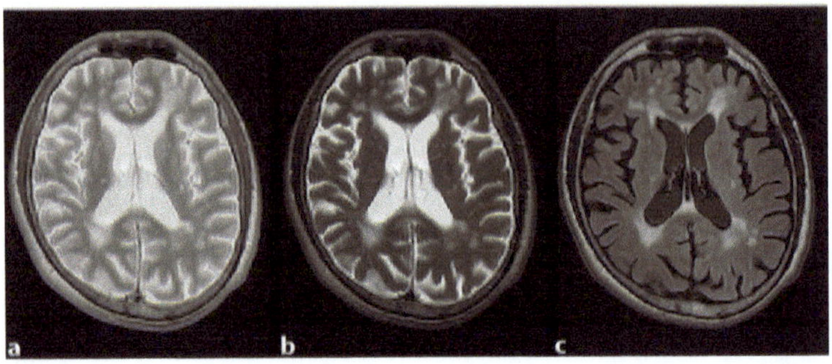

Fig. 5.1 Axial PD- (a), T2-weighted (b), and FLAIR (c) images of a patient with MS demonstrate enlargement of the ventricles and sulci, indicating brain atrophy. Note: Brain atrophy reflects the net result of the irreversible and destructive pathological process in MS. Gross morphological changes may be seen on standard magnetic resonance imaging and may appear more prominent on FLAIR sequences

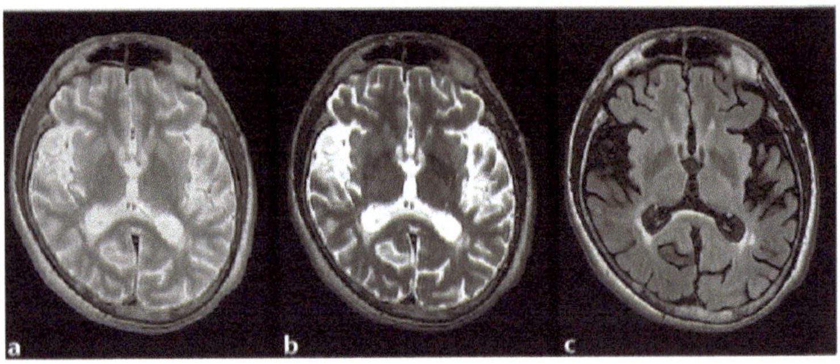

Fig. 5.2 Axial PD- (a), T2-weighted (b), and FLAIR (c) images of a patient with MS demonstrate severe brain atrophy, with enlargement of the ventricles. Note the enlargement of the third ventricle, severe atrophy of both temporal lobes, and prominent Sylvian fissures

5.3 Focal Atrophy

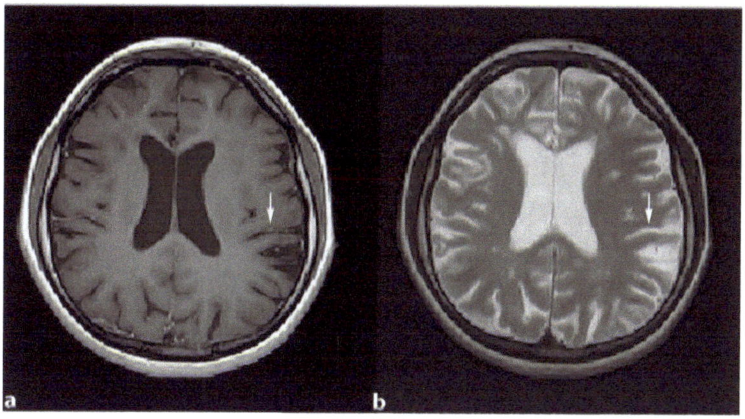

Fig. 5.3 Axial T1-weighted (**a**) and T2-weighted (**b**) images of a patient with MS demonstrate focal cortical atrophy (*arrows*). Note: Despite severe focal atrophy, there are only few MS lesions

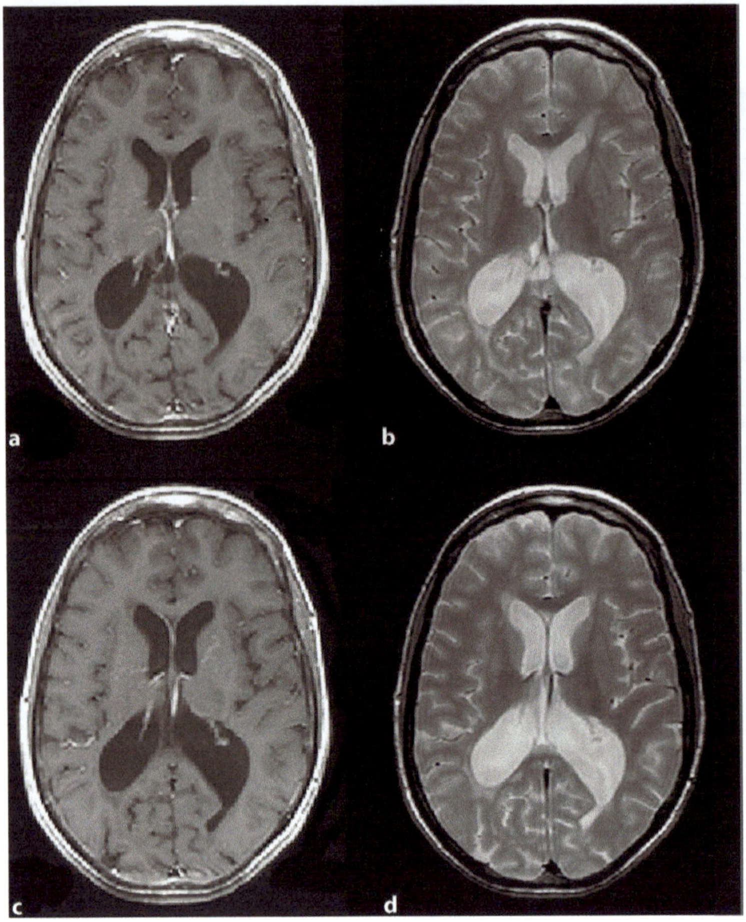

Fig. 5.4 Axial T1-weighted (**a,c**) and PD (**b,d**) images of a patient with MS demonstrate brain atrophy and severe ventricular enlargement, especially of the occipital horns. Note: There is no sign of decompensated hydrocephalus in this patient. Hydrocephalus in MS patients is due to tissue loss

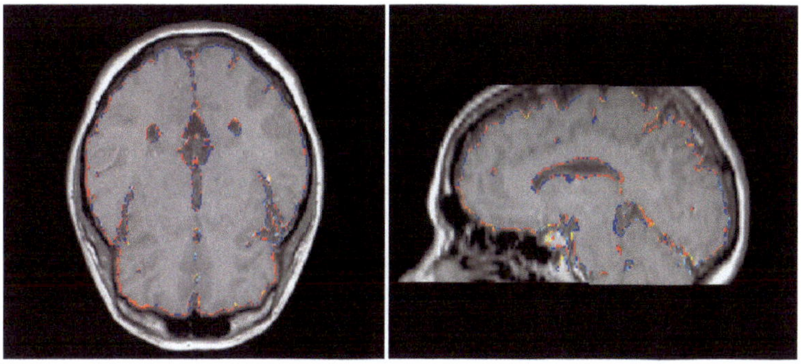

Fig. 5.5 Axial selected images of a patient with MS demonstrate measurement of brain atrophy with the structural image evaluation of normalised atrophy (SIENA) method. Note: Various methods have been prepared and implemented for analysis of brain atrophy. SIENA performs segmentation of brain from non-brain tissue in the head and registers two images to find atrophy. This method is used for longitudinal analysis

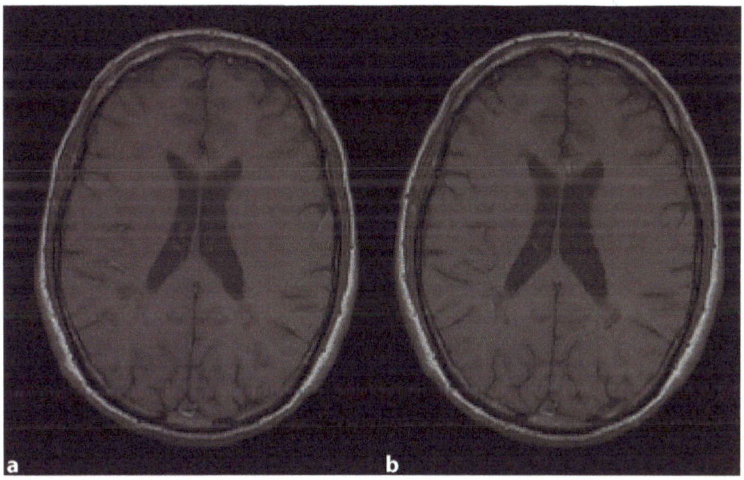

Fig. 5.6 Axial T1-weighted images at baseline (**a**) and after 1 year (**b**) have been used by the SIENA method to evaluate atrophy. This patient demonstrates a 2.1% brain volume loss in 1 year. The difference is not obvious if the images are observed with the eyes

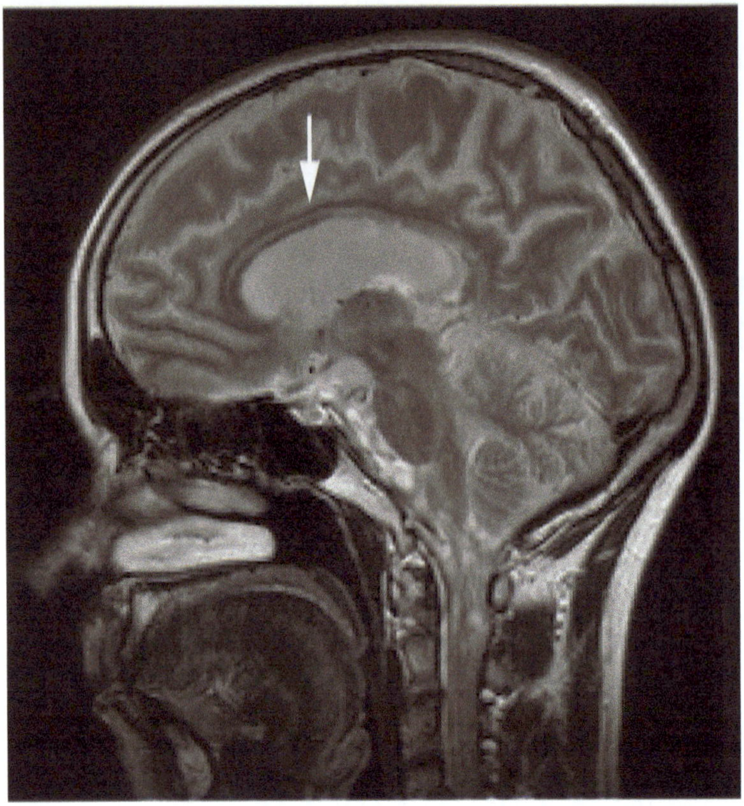

Fig. 5.7 Sagittal PD-weighted image of a patient with MS demonstrates thinning of the corpus callosum. Note: Diffuse or focal atrophy of the corpus callosum may be seen in later stages of MS

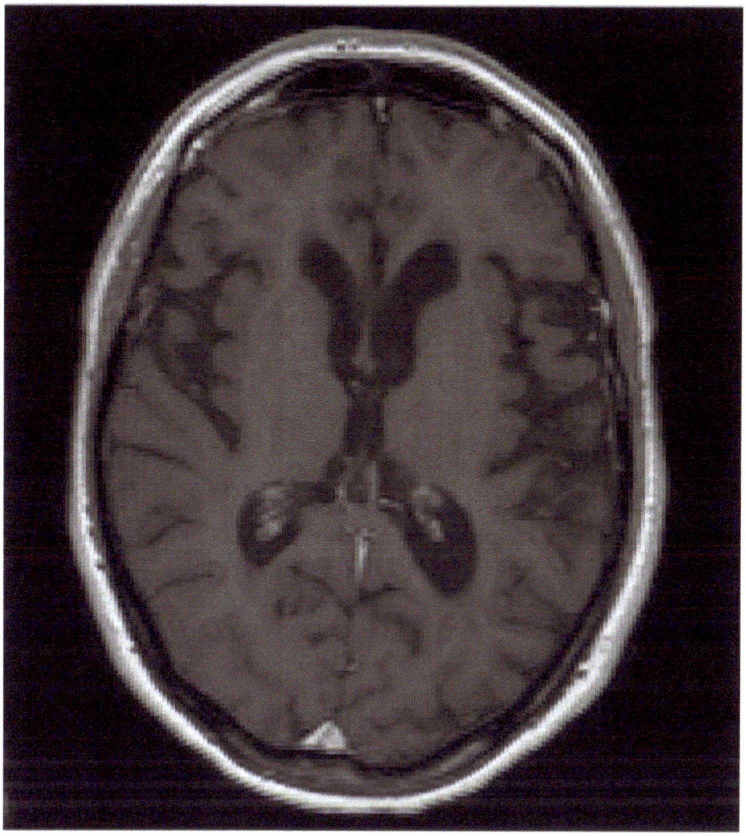

Fig. 5.8 Axial T1-weighted image of a patient with MS demonstrates ventricular dilatation and enlargement of the sulci especially in the left hemisphere

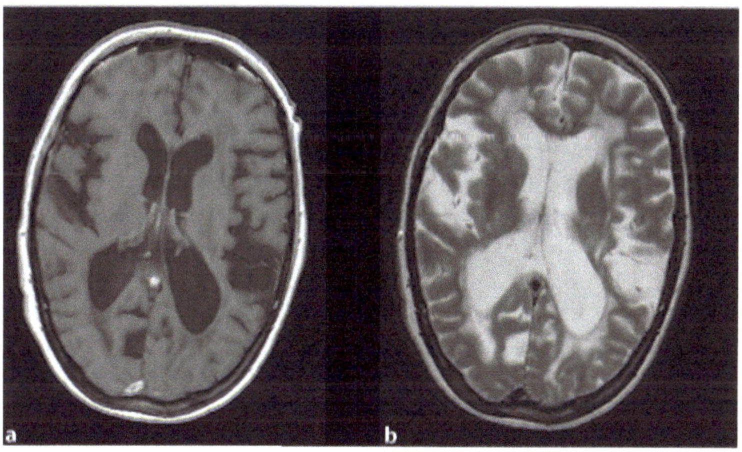

Fig. 5.9 Axial T1-weighted (**a**) and T2-weighted (**b**) images of a patient with secondary progressive MS demonstrate severe brain atrophy. Note: Secondary progressive MS (SPMS) may cause more atrophy than does RRMS

References

1. Benedict RH, Weinstock-Guttman B, Fishman I et al (2004) Prediction of neuropsychological impairment in multiple sclerosis: comparison of conventional magnetic resonance imaging measures of atrophy and lesion burden. Arch Neurol 6:226–230
2. Comi G, Rovaris M, Leocani L et al (2001) Clinical and MRI assessment of brain damage in MS. Neurol Sci 22(Suppl 2): S123–S127
3. Dastidar P, Heinonen T, Lehtimaki T et al (1999) Volumes of brain atrophy and plaques correlated with neurological disability in secondary progressive multiple sclerosis. J Neurol Sci 165:36–42
4. Fisher E, Rudick RA, Simon JH et al (2002) Eight-year follow-up study of brain atrophy in patients with MS. Neurology 59:1412–1420
5. Ge Y, Grossman RI, Udupa JK et al (2000) Brain atrophy in relapsing-remitting multiple sclerosis and secondary progressive multiple sclerosis: longitudinal quantitative analysis. Radiology 214:665–670
6. Hardmeier M, Wagenpfeil S, Freitag P, Fisher E, Rudick RA, Koojimans M, Clanet M, Radue EW, Kappos L; European Interferon Beta-1A in Relapsing MS Dose Comparison Trial Study Group (2003) Atrophy is detectable within a 3-month period in untreated patients with active relapsing remitting multiple sclerosis. Arch Neurol 60:1736–1739
7. Hardmeier M, Wagenpfeil S, Freitag P, Fisher E, Rudick RA, Koojimans M, Clanet M, Radue EW, Kappos L; European Interferon Beta-1A in Relapsing MS Dose Comparison Trial Study Group (2005) Rate of brain atrophy in relapsing MS decreases during treatment with IFN beta-1a. Neurology 64:236–240
8. Hardmeier M, Radue EW, Kappos L (2005) Short-term brain atrophy changes in relapsing-remitting multiple sclerosis (Letter to the Editor, article by Zivadinov et al). J Neurol Sci 231:101
9. Kalkers NF, Ameziane N, Bot JC et al (2002) Longitudinal brain volume measurement in multiple sclerosis: rate of brain atrophy is independent of the disease subtype. Arch Neurol 59:1572–1576
10. Losseff NA, Kingsley DP, McDonald WI et al (1996) Clinical and magnetic resonance imaging predictors of disability in primary and secondary progressive multiple sclerosis. Mult Scler 1:218–222
11. Miller DH, Barkhof F, Frank JA (2002) Measurement of atrophy in multiple sclerosis: pathological basis, methodological aspects and clinical relevance. Brain 125:1676–1695
12. Paolillo A, Pozzilli C, Gasperini C et al (2000) Brain atrophy in relapsing-remitting multiple sclerosis: relationship with "black holes," disease duration and clinical disability. J Neurol Sci 174:85–91
13. Rovaris M, Comi G, Rocca MA et al (2001) Short-term brain volume change in relapsing-remitting multiple sclerosis: effect of glatiramer acetate and implications. Brain 124:1803–1812
14. Rudick RA (2004) Impact of disease-modifying therapies on brain and spinal cord atrophy in multiple sclerosis J Neuroimaging 14(3 Suppl):S54–S64
15. Zivadinov R, Bakshi R (2004) Role of MRI in multiple sclerosis II: brain and spinal cord atrophy. Front Biosci 9:647–664
16. Zivadinov R, Zorzon M (2004) Is gadolinium enhancement predictive of the development of brain atrophy in multiple sclerosis? A review of the literature J Neuroimaging 12:302–309
17. Zivadinov R, Sepcic J, Nasuelli D et al (2001) A longitudinal study of brain atrophy and cognitive disturbances in the early phase of relapsing-remitting multiple sclerosis. J Neurol Neurosurg Psychiatry 70:773–780

6 Pitfalls in the Depiction of MS Lesions on Conventional MRI

M.A. Sahraian, E.-W. Radue

6.1 Introduction

New data emphasize early diagnosis and treatment with available disease-modifying therapies in MS (Rieckmam 2005), but establishing the diagnosis of MS is not always a straightforward process, and many other inflammatory and noninflammatory neurological diseases can mimic MS on neuroimaging or clinical presentation (Charil et al. 2006).

We discuss the differential diagnosis of MS in a separate chapter, and demonstrate several images on this issue (see Chap. 9). However, another point of importance is that some normal anatomical structures or artifacts may mimic MS plaques on MRI. Regarding the new diagnostic criteria, MRI plays an important role in the diagnosis of MS and the depiction of a new lesion may fulfill the criteria (Polman et al. 2005) (see Chap. 8). Correct identification and differentiation of the lesions from normal structures are therefore mandatory and prevent wrong diagnosis in suspected cases.

Anatomical structures that may generate pitfalls in MR images include CSF-containing structures, enhancing vessels, and partial volume effect of ventricles or gray matter.

The following hints are advised for interpretation of suspected lesions:

1. Look at serial slices above and below the images.
2. Look at other sequences to compare the intensity of lesions in T2 long, PD, and FLAIR.
3. Look at previous examinations and especially compare MRI parameters.
4. Consider follow-up examinations in suspected cases.
5. For follow-up images always use the same parameters as baseline. Changing parameters (echo time, echo train) may result in different intensities as compared with previous examination(s).
6. Try to cover the whole brain so that the lesions in the vertex or lower parts of the brainstem are not missed. A standard MRI with 3-mm slice thickness without any gap between them is advised (Simon et al. 2006).
7. Image repositioning should be compared to the baseline scan.

Another pitfall in the interpretation of brain or spinal cord MRI is missing the lesions that result in false-negative reports. It should be noted that MS is basically a clinical diagnosis, and MRI should not be interpreted without considering the clinical history of the patients (Schiffer et al. 1993).

This chapter deals with the above-mentioned problems in depicting MS lesions and demonstrates examples of artifacts and normal anatomical structures that may mimic MS plaques.

6.2 Virchow-Robin Spaces

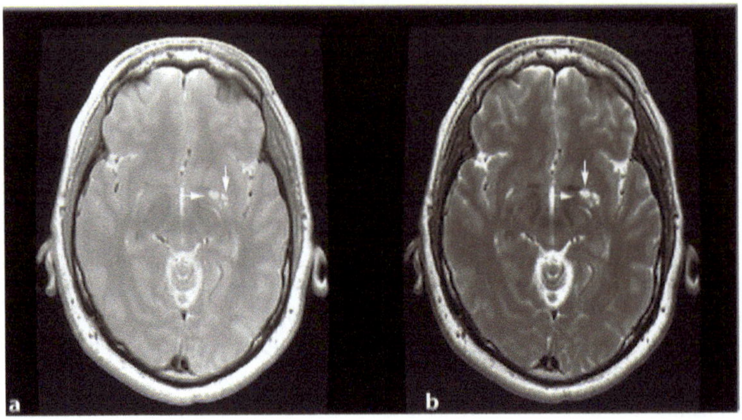

Fig. 6.1 Axial (**a**) and T2-weighted (**b**) images of a patient with RRMS demonstrate Virchow-Robin spaces (*arrows*). Note: Virchow-Robin spaces are perivascular spaces that surround small arteries and arterioles as they perforate the surface of the brain and extend into the brain tissue. These CSF-containing structures may dilate and mimic MS lesions

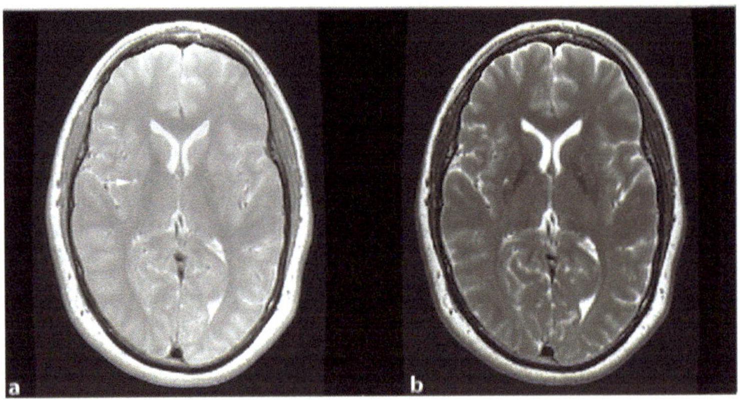

Fig. 6.2 Axial PD- (**a**) and T2-weighted (**b**) images of a patient with MS demonstrate a Virchow-Robin space in the right putamen (*arrow*). Note: The basal ganglia and the corona radiata are common sites for dilated Virchow-Robin spaces

6.3 Vessels: Arteries

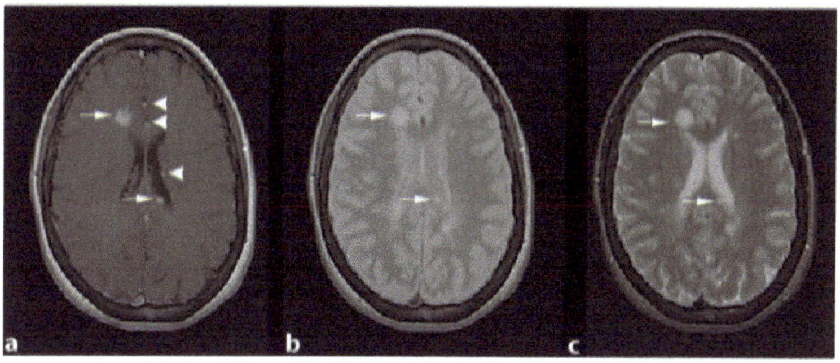

Fig. 6.3 Axial T1-weighted with contrast (**a**), PD- (**b**), and T2-weighted (**c**) images of a patient with MS demonstrate two enhancing lesions (*arrows*) and three enhancing vessels (*arrowheads*). Note: Enhancing vessels may be mistaken as Gd enhancing lesions. Consider that almost all enhancing lesions have corresponding T2 abnormalities, and enhancing vessels are usually iso- or hypointense on T2-weighted images

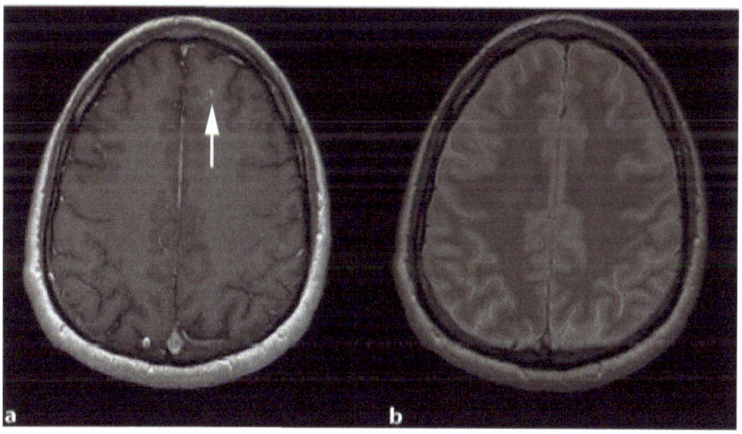

Fig. 6.4 Axial T1-weighted with contrast (**a**) and PD (**b**) images demonstrate an enhancing structure (*arrow*) without corresponding T2 abnormalities, which seems to be a vessel

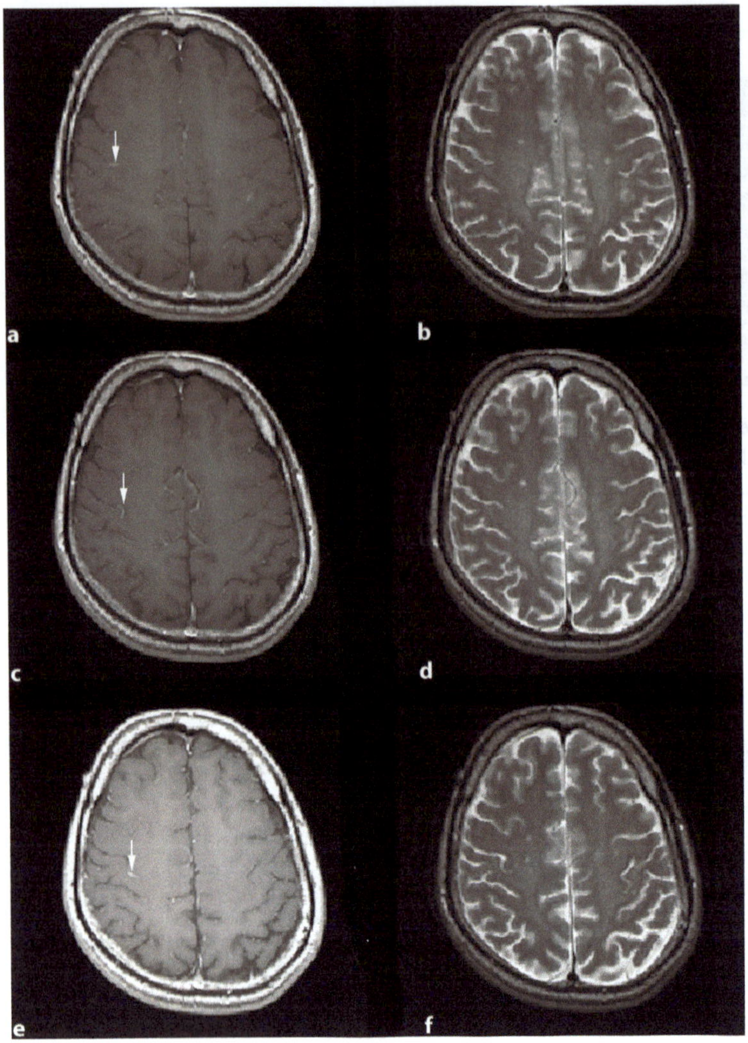

Fig. 6.5 Axial T1-weighted with contrast (**a,c,e**) and T2-weighted (**b,d,f**) images demonstrate an enhancing vessel (*arrows*). Note: There is no corresponding abnormality on the T2-weighted images. The consecutive slices show that the hyperintense structure follows the shape of a vascular structure. Observation of upper and lower slices and different sequences is valuable to differentiate real plaques from non–MS pathologies or normal structures

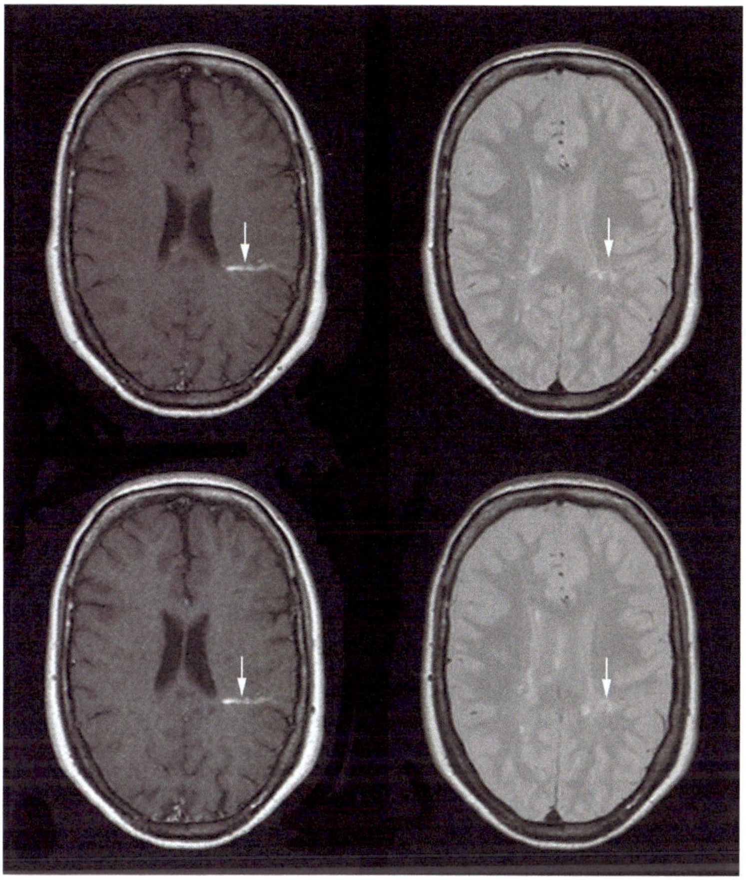

Fig. 6.6 Axial T1-weighted with contrast and PD images of a patient with MS at baseline (*upper images*) and after 1 year (*lower images*) demonstrate an enhancing vessel with corresponding T2 abnormality. Note: Enhancing structures that persist more than 6 months are more likely to be vascular structures. Most MS lesions lose their enhancement within 3 months

6.4 Vessels: Veins

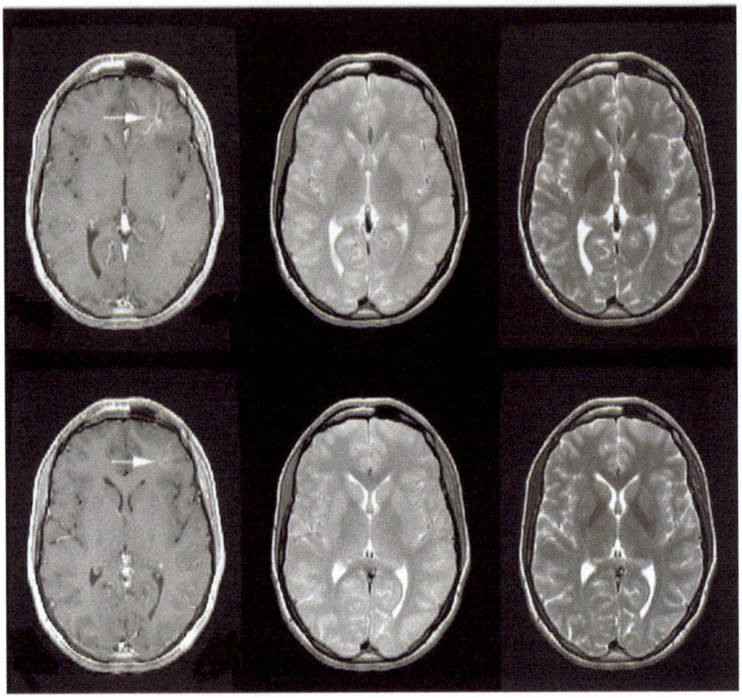

Fig. 6.7 Axial T1-weighted with contrast, PD-, and T2-weighted images of a patient with MS demonstrate an enhancing vascular structure (venous angioma) in two consecutive slices (*arrows*). The abnormality may mimic an enhancing MS plaque if just one slice is observed (T1-weighted in *lower row*), but looking at other slices and sequences helps in differentiation

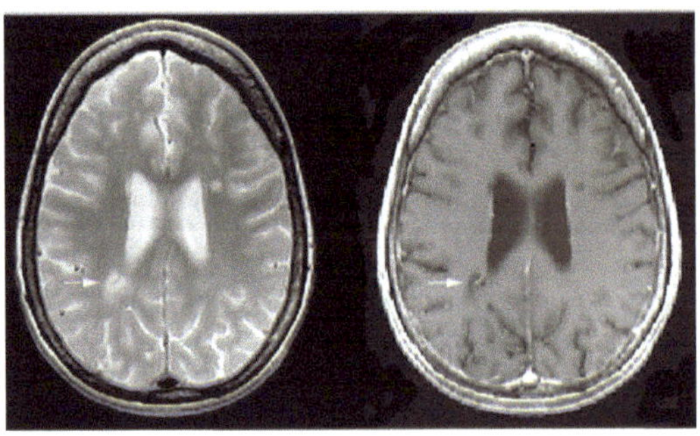

Fig. 6.8 Axial T2-weighted and T1-weigthed with contrast images demonstrate a hyperintense T2-weighted lesion with its corresponding black hole and a hypointense central venous structure (*arrows*). The enhancing vessel inside the lesion should not be mistaken as a partial enhancement of the lesion. Note the corresponding T2 hypointensity inside the lesion

6.5 Partial Volume Effect: Ventricular Caps

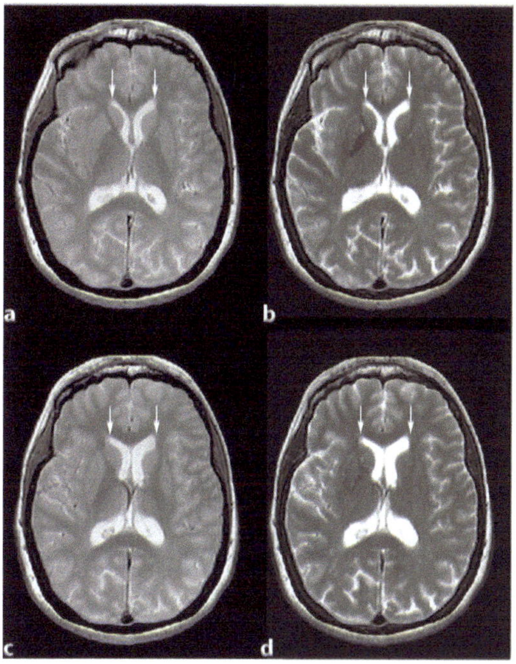

Fig. 6.9 Axial PD- (a,c) and T2-weigthed (**b,d**) images of a patient with MS demonstrate slight hyperintensity attached to the frontal horns of the lateral ventricles (ventricular caps) (*arrows*). Note: High signal intensity around the pole of the frontal horns (caps) is particularly common and is due to an age-related focal loss of ependyma with subependymal gliosis, leading to an increased water content

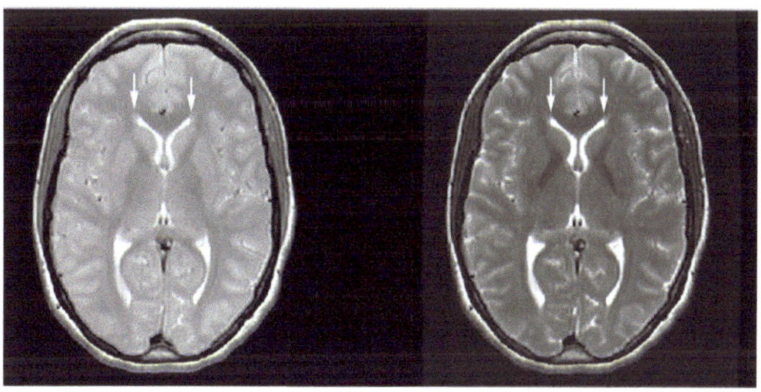

Fig. 6.10 Axial PD- and T2-weighted images demonstrate ventricular caps that may be mistaken as lesions (*arrows*)

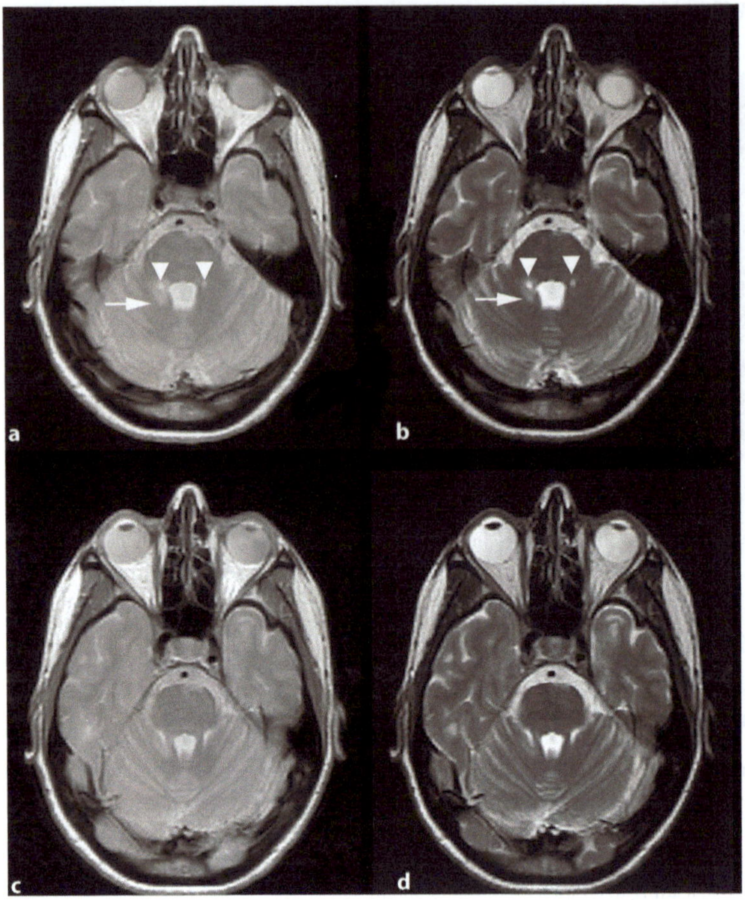

Fig. 6.11 Axial PD- (**a**) and T2-weighted (**b**) images of a patient with RRMS demonstrate a lesion attached to the 4th ventricle (*arrows*). The symmetrical hyperintensities on both sides of the 4th ventricle are partial volume effects of the cisterns (*arrowheads*). The upper slices (**c**,**d**) demonstrate the cisterns. Note: Partial volume effects of the cisterns may mimic MS lesions. Special attention should be given to the upper and lower slices

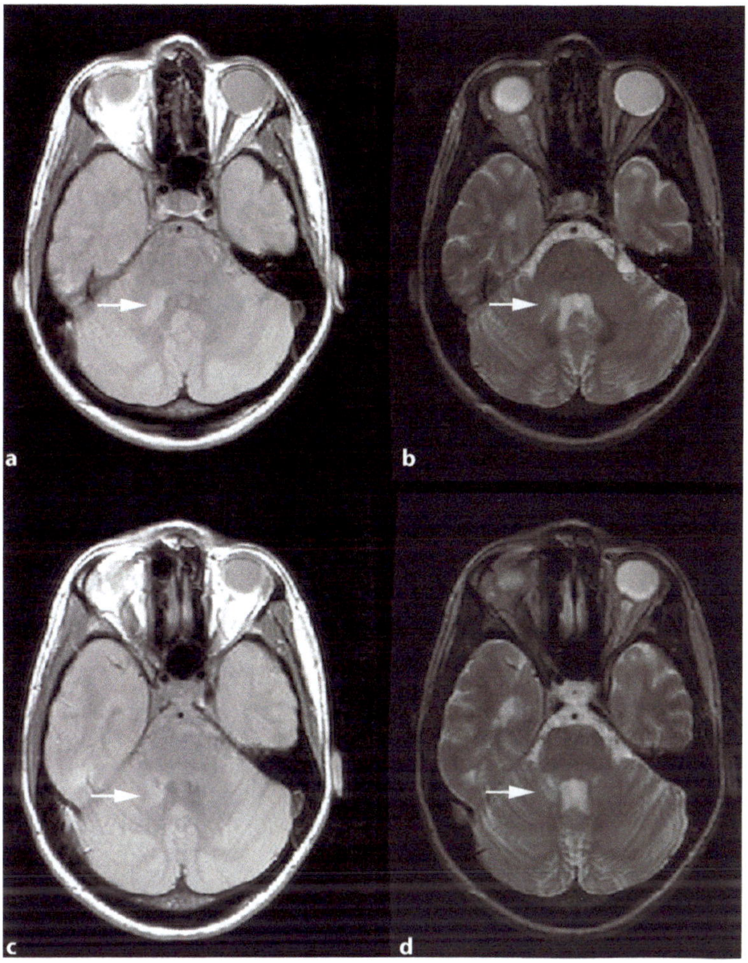

Fig. 6.12 Axial PD- (**a**,**c**) and T2-weighted (**b**,**d**) images of a patient with RRMS demonstrate a lesion attached to the 4th ventricle (*arrows*). Note the partial volume effect of the peripontine cistern inside the lesion

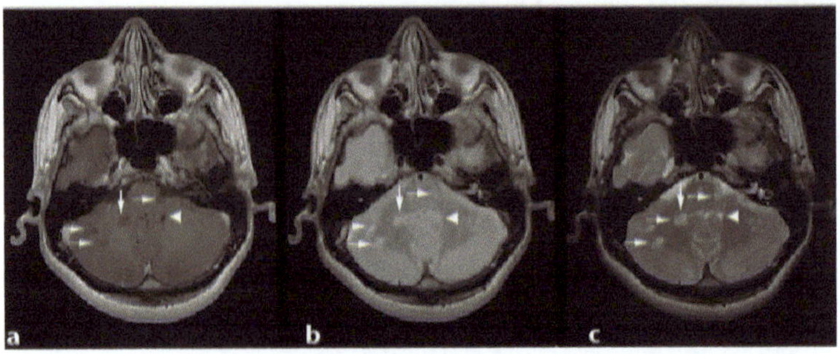

Fig. 6.13 Axial T1-weighted with contrast (**a**), PD- (**b**), and T2-weighted images (**c**) demonstrate several black holes in the posterior fossa with their corresponding T2 abnormalities (*arrows*). The partial volume effect of the 4th ventricle in the T1-weighted image (*arrowheads*) should not be taken as a lesion. Comparison with other sequences will help in differentiation

6.6 Artifacts

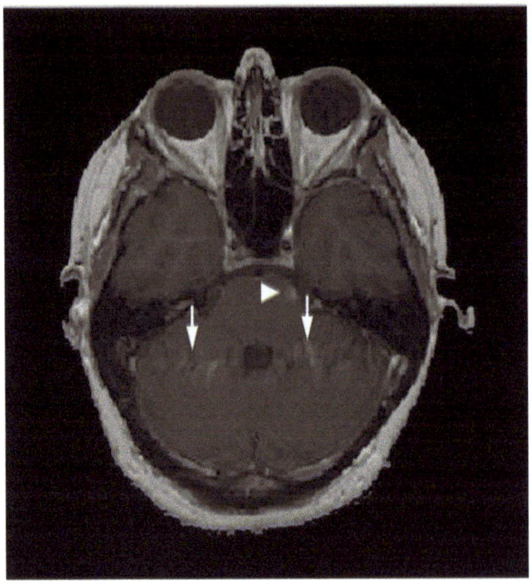

Fig. 6.14 Axial T1-weighted image with contrast demonstrates an artifact in the posterior fossa passing through the 4th ventricle (*arrow*). An enhancing lesion of the pons is also seen in this image (*arrowhead*)

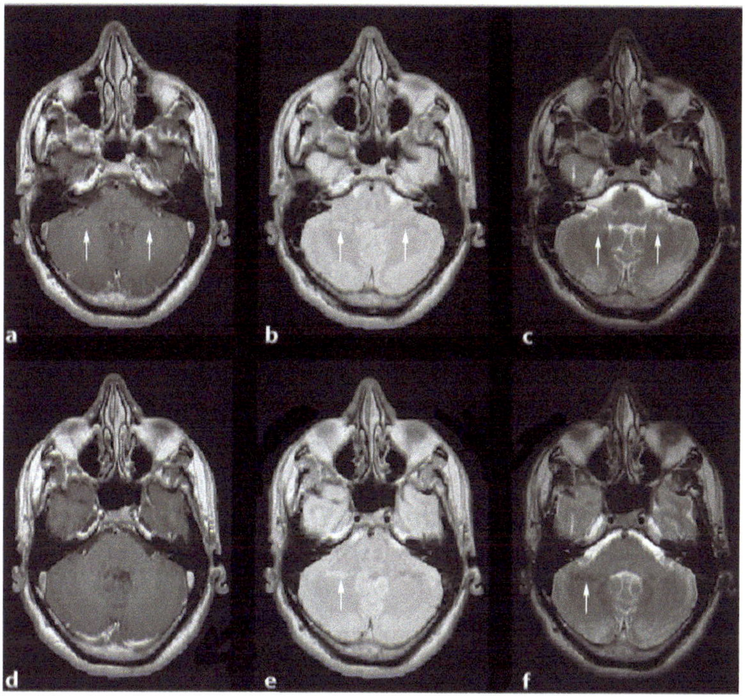

Fig. 6.15 Axial T1-weighted with contrast (**a**,**d**), PD- (**b**,**e**), and T2-weighted (**c**,**f**) images of a patient with MS demonstrate a line of artifact passing through the 4th ventricle. Note: Artifacts in the posterior fossa may induce hyperintensities that should not be mistaken as lesions. Comparison with other sequences will help in differentiation

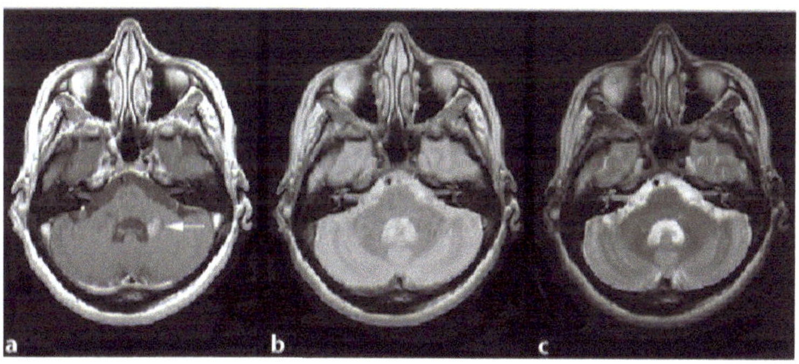

Fig. 6.16 Axial T1-weighted with contrast (**a**), PD- (**b**), and T2-weighted (**c**) images of a patient with MS demonstrate an artifact near the 4th ventricle (*arrow*). Note: Lack of a corresponding T2 abnormality and the artifact line that is visible on the left side of the 4th ventricle help in differentiation

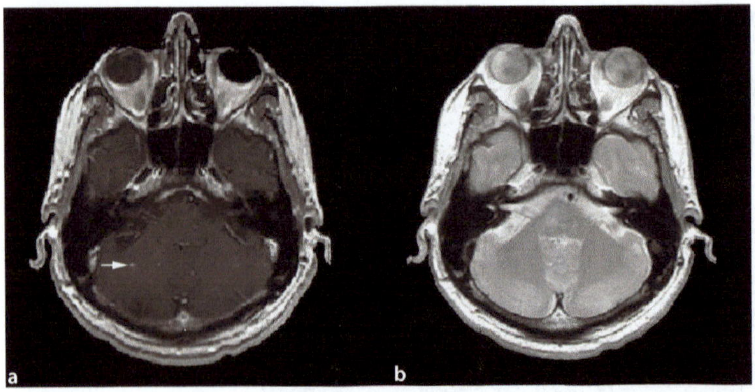

Fig. 6.17 Axial T1-weighted with contrast (**a**) and corresponding PD (**b**) images demonstrate an artifact in the left cerebellar hemisphere (*arrow*), which may be mistaken as an enhancing lesion. Absence of any corresponding T2 abnormality helps in differentiation

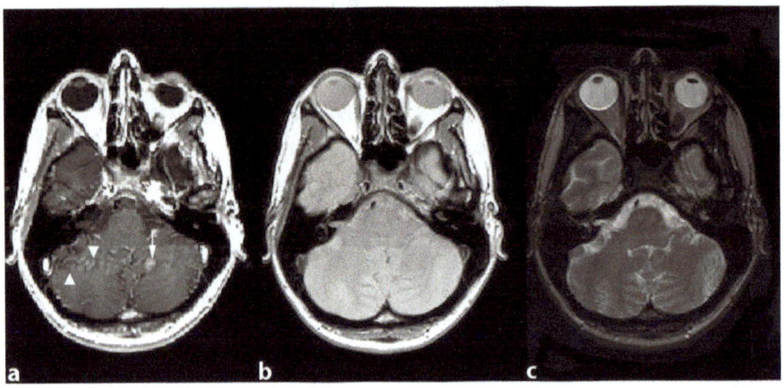

Fig. 6.18 Axial T1-weighted with contrast (**a**), corresponding PD- (**b**), and T2-weighted (**c**) images of a patient with RRMS demonstrate a hyperintensity in the left cerebellar hemisphere (*arrow*) without corresponding T2 abnormality that may be mistaken as a MS lesion. Look at the artifact line over the cerebellum (*arrowheads*)

6.7 Special Locations

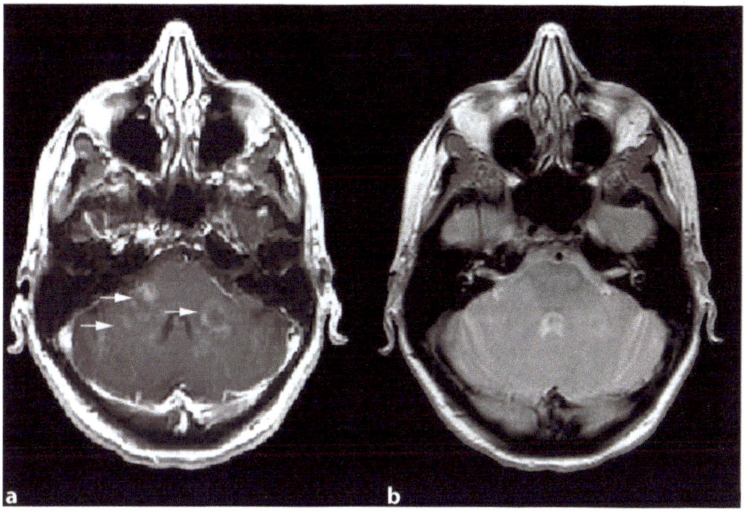

Fig. 6.19 Axial T1-weighted with contrast (**a**) and PD (**b**) and images of a patient with RRMS demonstrate several artifacts in the cerebellar hemispheres and peduncles (*arrows*)

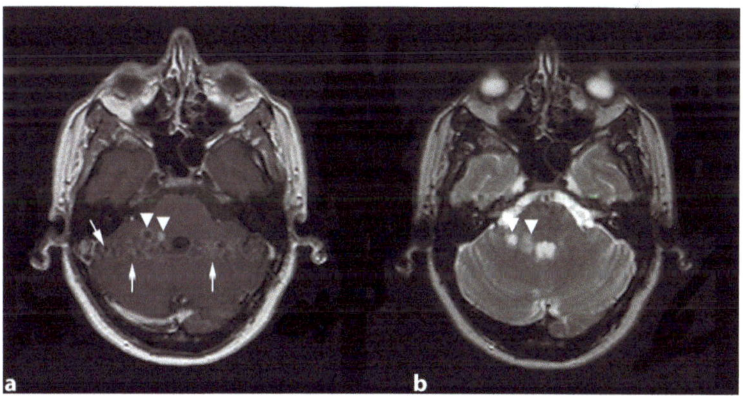

Fig. 6.20 Axial T1-weighted with contrast (**a**) and PD (**b**) images demonstrate an artifact line in the posterior fossa passing through the 4th ventricle (*arrows*). Two Gd enhancing lesions (ring type and nodular type) are exactly above the artifacts. The lesions may be missed due to the artifact (*arrowheads*)

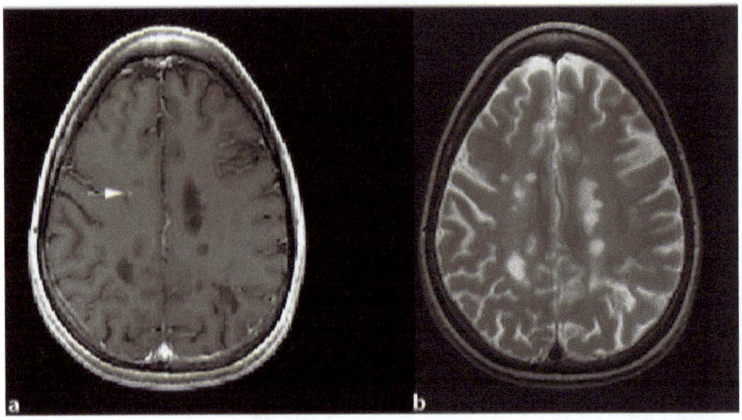

Fig. 6.21 Axial T2-weighted with contrast (a) and corresponding T2-weighted (b) images demonstrate a small enhancing lesion. Such lesions may be easily missed if the images are not reviewed carefully

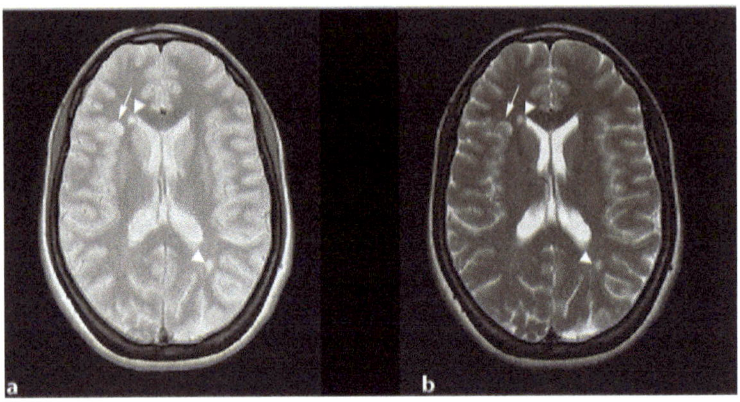

Fig. 6.22 Axial PD- (a) and T2-weighted (b) images demonstrate a juxtacortical lesion (*arrows*). This lesion may be easily missed on the long T2-weighted image. Other lesions are demonstrated by *arrowheads*

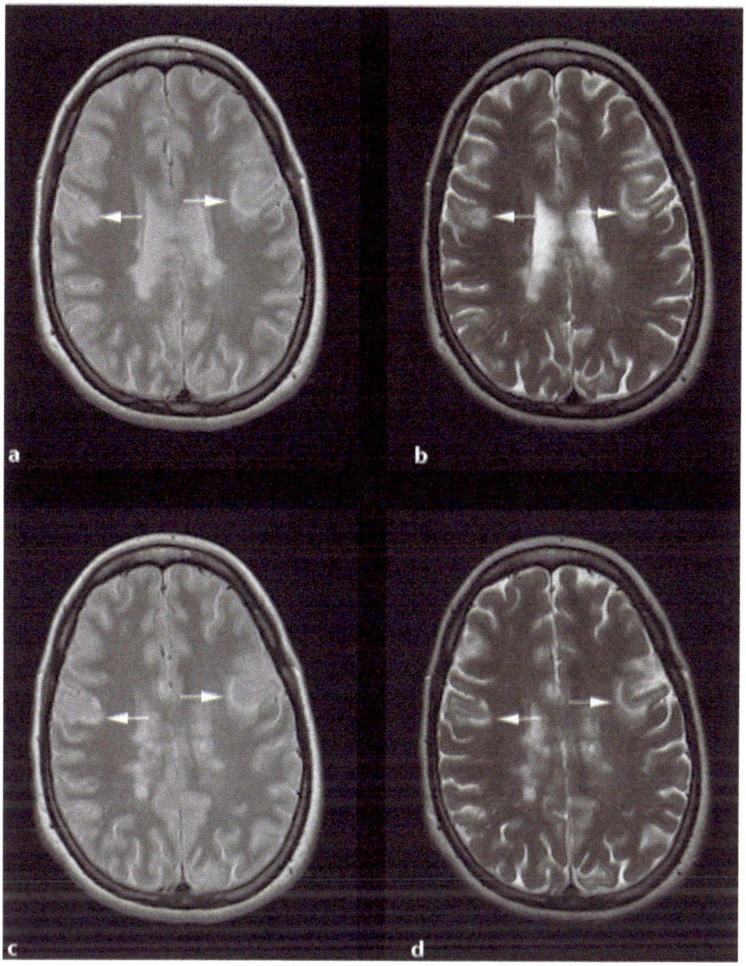

Fig. 6.23 Axial PD- (a,c) and T2-weighted (**b**,**d**) images of a patient with RRMS demonstrate several MS lesions. The lesions in **b** (*arrows*) may be missed if upper slices or the corresponding PD are not observed carefully

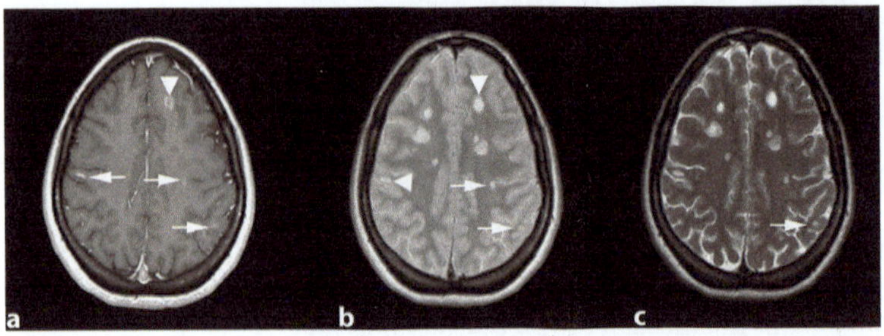

Fig. 6.24 Axial T1-weighted with contrast (**a**), PD- (**b**), and T2-weighted (**c**) images of a patient with MS demonstrate several enhancing lesions with their corresponding abnormalities. The enhancing lesion in the left frontal lobe (*arrowhead*) is clear, but other enhancing lesions may be missed if the sequences are not compared with the corresponding T2-weighted image (*arrows*)

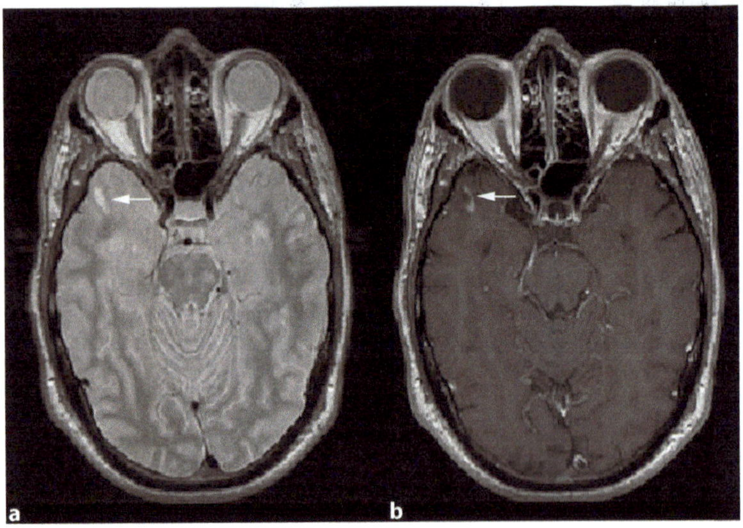

Fig. 6.25 Axial PD- (**a**) and T1-weighted images with contrast (**b**) demonstrate a juxtacortical enhancing lesion in the temporal lobe (*arrows*). Note: Lesions in the temporal lobes especially the temporal poles may be missed if the images are not observed and different sequences are not carefully compared

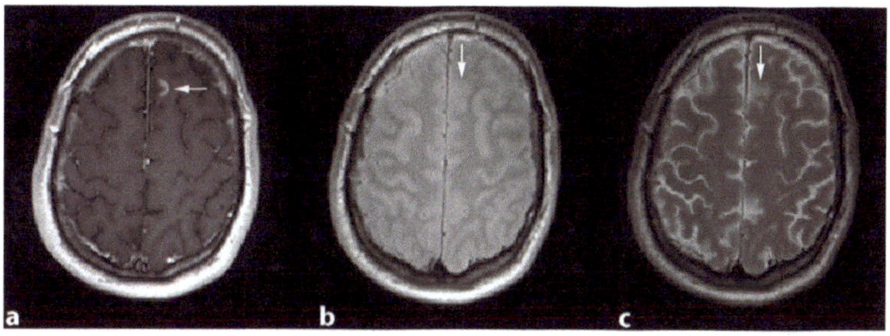

Fig. 6.26 Axial T1-weighted with contrast (**a**), PD- (**b**), and T2-weighted images demonstrate a cortical/subcortical enhancing lesion. Note: The lesion is iso- or slightly hyperintense on PD and may be missed if other sequences are ignored

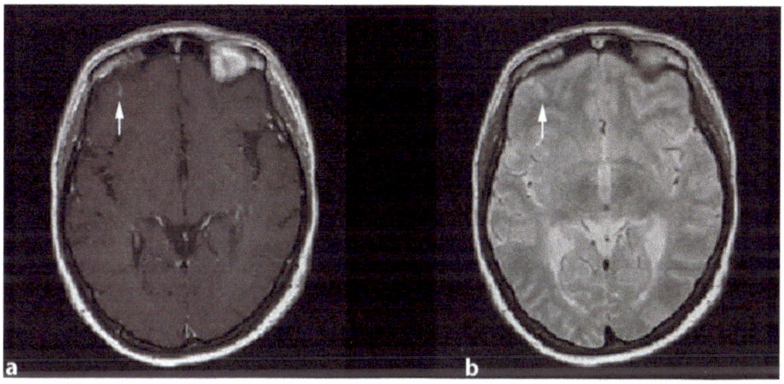

Fig. 6.27 Axial T1-weighted with contrast (**a**) and PD (**b**) images demonstrate an enhancing lesion in the left frontal lobe that may be missed if the two sequences are not compared

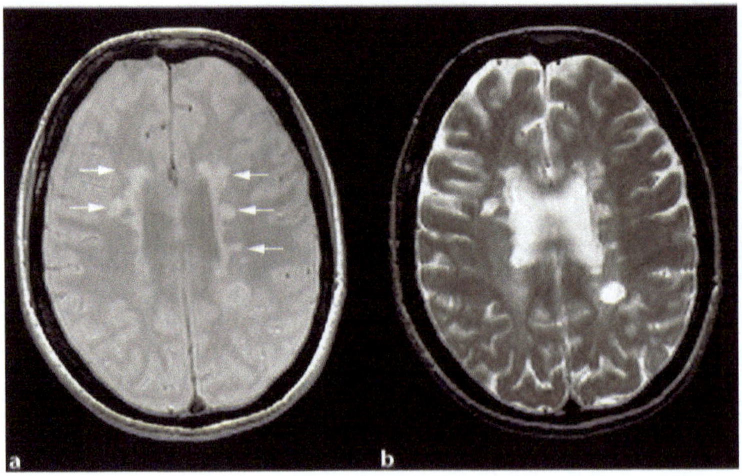

Fig. 6.28 Axial PD- (a) and T2-weighted (b) images of a patient with RRMS demonstrate periventricular MS lesions (*arrows*). Note: MS lesions may be missed in T2-weighted images due to CSF hyperintensity. PD images with special parameters or FLAIR are preferred for periventricular lesions

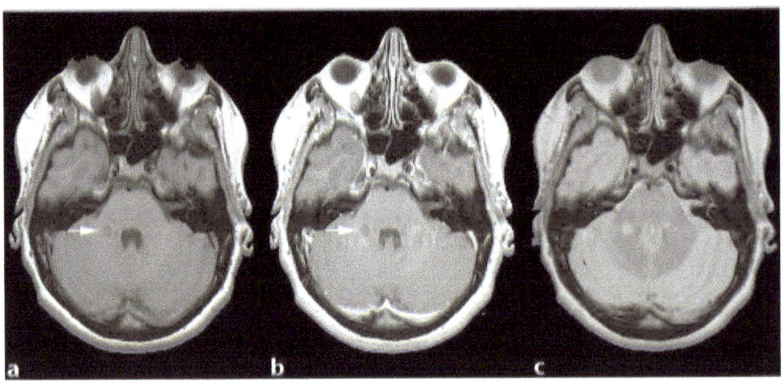

Fig. 6.29 Axial T1-weighted without (a), with contrast (b), and PD (c) images demonstrate a lesion in the left cerebellar peduncle. A line of artifact passes over it, and the lesion looks like an enhancing one, but comparison with the T1-without-Gd sequence shows that the lesion is non-enhancing (*arrows*)

References

1. Charil A, Yousry TA, Rovaris M et al (2006) MRI and the diagnosis of multiple sclerosis: expanding the concept of "no better explanation." Lancet Neurol 5:841–852
2. Rieckmann P (2005) Neurodegeneration and clinical relevance for early treatment in multiple sclerosis. Int MS J 12:42–51
3. Schiffer RB, Giang DW, Mushlin A et al (1993). Perils and pitfalls of magnetic resonance imaging in the diagnosis of multiple sclerosis. The Rochester-Toronto MRI Study Group. J Neuroimag 3:81–88
4. Simon JH, Li D, Traboulsee A et al (2006) Standardized MR imaging protocol for multiple sclerosis: Consortium of MS Centers consensus guidelines. AJNR Am J Neuroradiol 27:455-461

7 Magnetic Resonance Imaging of the Spinal Cord in Multiple Sclerosis

K. Weier, S. Haller, A. Gass

7.1 Introduction

Although the spinal cord is frequently involved in MS, up to now MRI of the cord is only performed for a number of special indications. In particular, it is rarely performed as a screening examination together with MRI of the brain. Due to the small cord size, high spatial resolution is needed on MRI. The mobility of the cord is a problem, and surrounding tissue as well as CSF pulsation and cardiac or respiratory motions can cause artifacts, which sometimes unpredictably can reduce image quality. Spinal cord imaging has improved considerably with the use of phased array coils, and recently parallel imaging has improved time efficiency of cord MRI.

The spinal cord is usually assessed in the sagittal plane, which allows a fairly quick reference, but is an unusual plane when detailed visualization of an anatomical structure is the aim. A second plane is state of the art for the detailed visualization of the cord cross-section, as is shown in most of the illustrations of this chapter. Previous and current studies have shown that in up to 90% of patients with definite MS spinal cord changes can be detected and appear either as focal lesions, diffuse abnormalities or as a combination of both (Figs. 7.1–7.4).

Atrophy of the cord over small segments or even of the whole cord is a common long-term sequela in MS patients and can be detected by MRI (Figs. 7.5, 7.6).

From the neuropathologist's view, histopathological analysis shows focal lesions that are sharply delineated and can be found at all levels of the cord but are more frequently seen in cervical parts. They are usually multiple in number (mean: 3 to 4) and approximately one to two vertebras in length (Bot et al. 2004; Kidd et al. 1993).

Diffuse histopathological changes are observed as an area of increased signal intensity and are best seen on PD-weighted scans (Lycklama et al. 2003). The diffuse hyperintensity on MRI is characterized by a not-well-demarcated abnormality consisting of some degree of demyelination and axonal loss, affecting the entire diameter and usually involving several segments in length. Additional axial images can help to characterize changes that are not obviously seen on the sagittal images and can confirm or reject subtle changes.

Plaques in the spinal cord tend to be located in the periphery of the cord and usually do not respect the boundaries between gray and white matter (Adams et al. 1952; Tartaglino et al. 1995) (Figs. 7.2, 7.3). Most commonly, the demyelination affects the dorsolateral aspects of the cord. Acute lesions are often associated with cord swelling and may show contrast enhancement on T1-weighted images (Figs. 7.7, 7.8). Compared with brain MRI T1 hypointense lesions (black holes) are rarely described in the spinal cord (Gass et al. 1998), probably due to its compact tissue organization. It has been shown that MRI signal abnormalities in the spinal cord are more specific for MS, compared with brain T2-hyperintensities (Thorpe 1993). Cord lesions due to microangiopathy have not been reported, and therefore the prevalence of asymptomatic cord lesions in patients over the age of 50 is lower than it is in the brain. A positive MRI therefore is often suggestive of an inflammatory–demyelinating disease.

This chapter illustrates the most important MRI morphological features of MS lesions.

7.2 Lesions

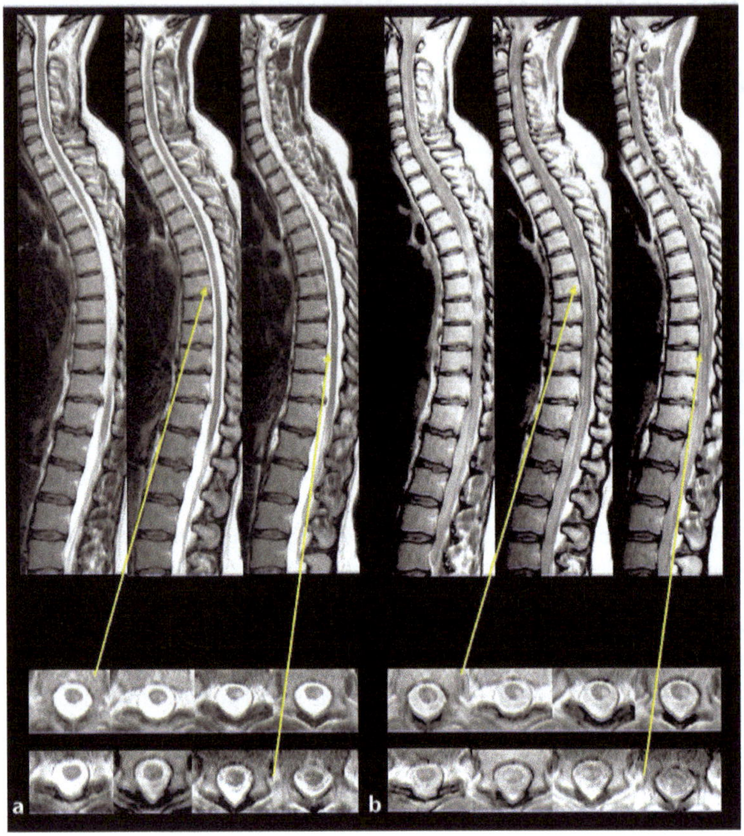

Fig. 7.1 Sagittal and transverse T2- (**a**) and PD-weighted (**b**) images of the spinal cord. The T2-weighted images allow differentiation of the cord from CSF and demonstrate hyperintense lesions that are more strongly contrasted on the PD-weighted slices, while the differentiation of the cord from the CSF is more difficult. The combination of the two contrasts is helpful to delineate anatomical features and lesions (*yellow arrows*). The transverse plane allows localization of the lesions with respect to their cross-sectional extent

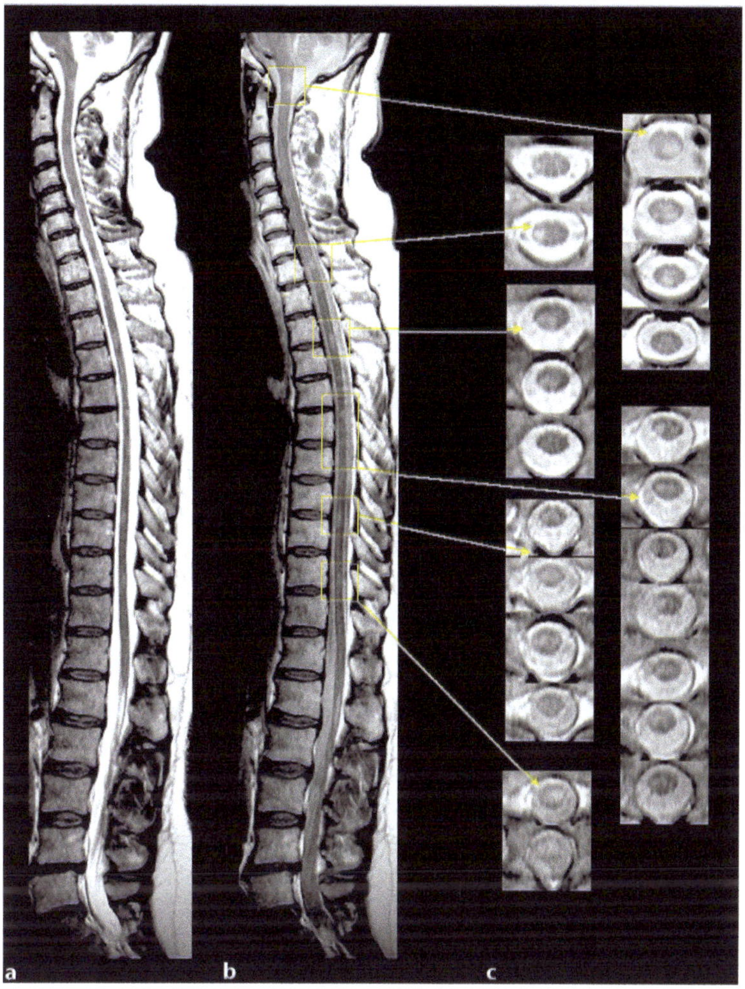

Fig. 7.2 T2- (a) and proton density-weighted (b,c) images of the entire cord-showing typical focal lesions at several cord levels. Corresponding T2-hyperintense lesions are noted at respective levels demonstrating thelocation and extent of the lesion in the cross-sectional perspective

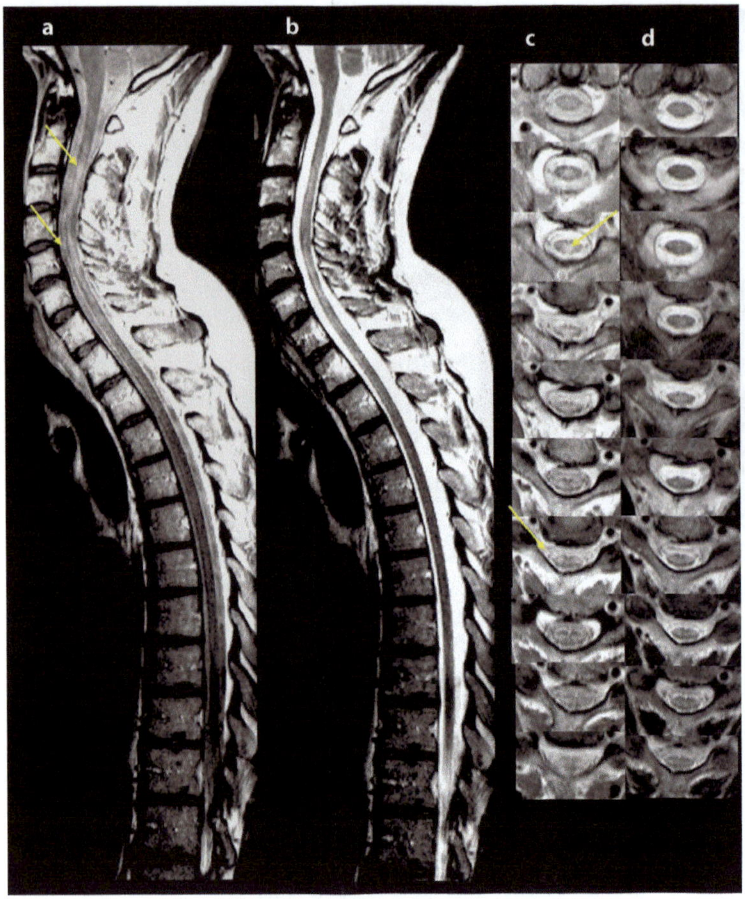

Fig. 7.3 Sagittal and transverse PD- (**a**,**c**) and T2-weighted (**b**,**d**) images of the whole cord, demonstrating both focal and diffuse changes. Multiple lesions are seen at the cervical and upper thoracic cord. Besides the obvious hyperintense lesions, focal atrophy of the cord is appreciated

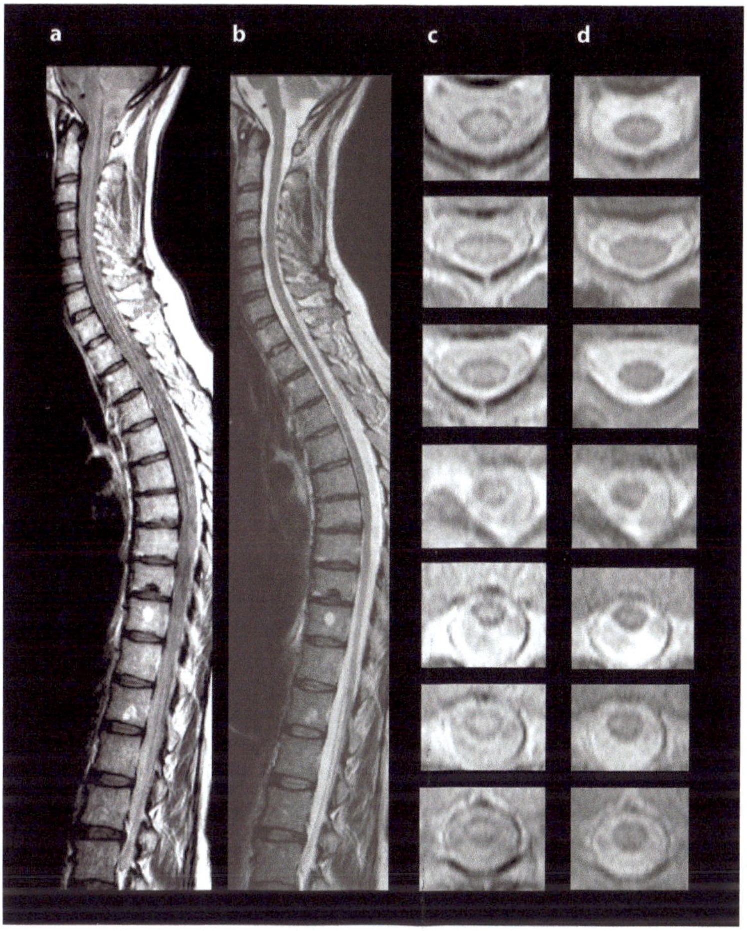

Fig. 7.4 Sagittal and transverse PD- (**a**,**c**) and T2-weighted (**b**,**d**) images of the whole cord. Diffuse abnormalities can be seen along the whole length of the cord and are shown with strong contrast on the PD-weighted images. The transverse images also show some diffuse hyperintensity affecting the cross-section of the cord

7.3 Atrophy

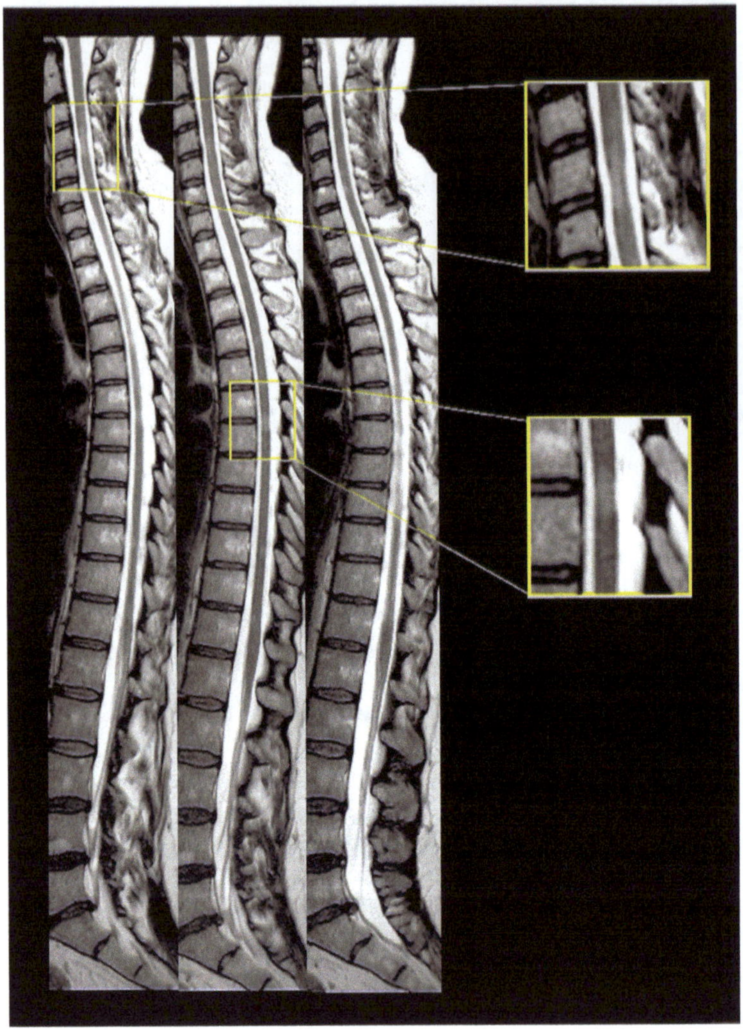

Fig. 7.5 Sagittal T2-weighted images of the spinal cord. Focal atrophy is shown in magnification as characteristic residual signs of chronic cord changes

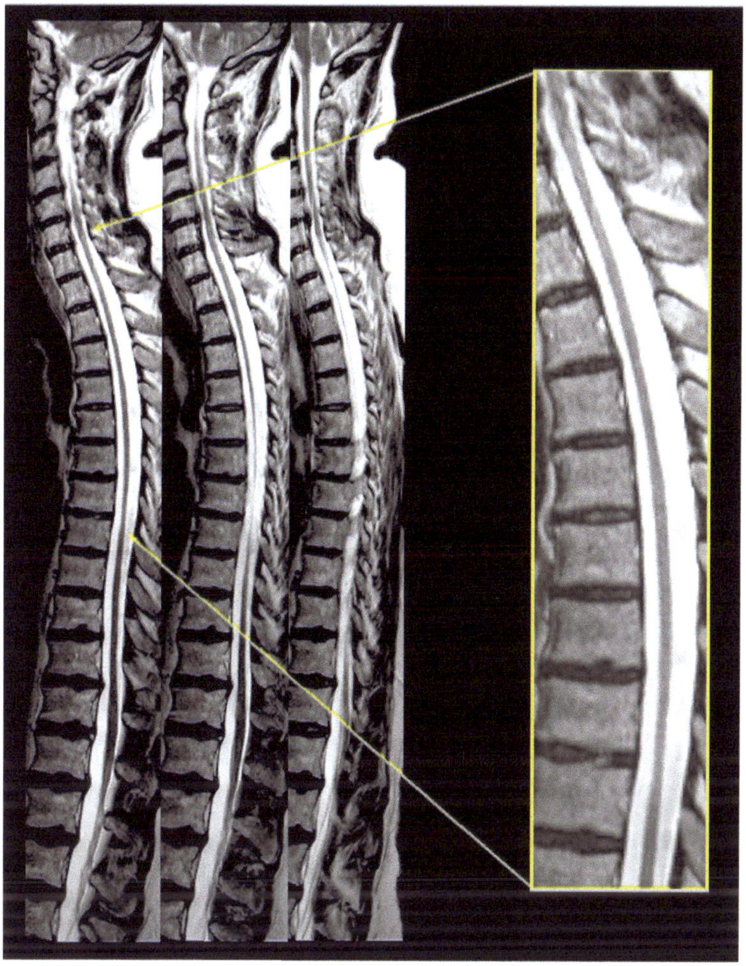

Fig. 7.6 Sagittal T2-weighted images of the spinal cord. Residual multisegmental cord atrophy as a typical sign of chronic tissue destruction is shown in magnification

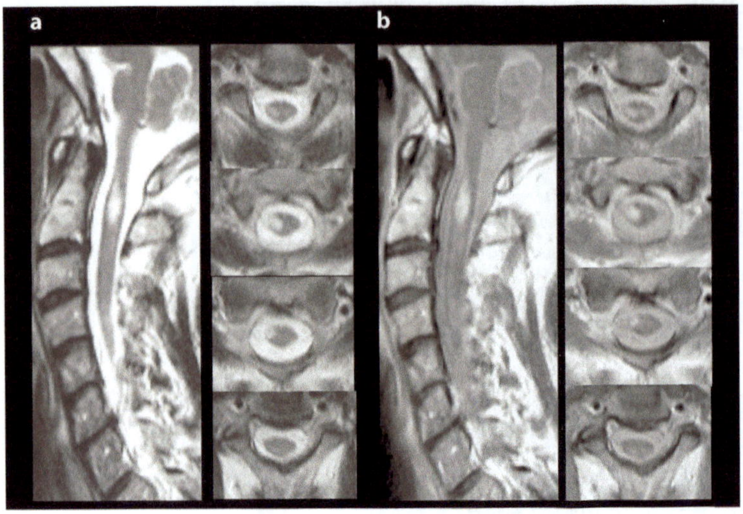

Fig. 7.7 Sagittal and transverse T2-weighted (**a**) and PD (**b**) images of the cervical cord, demonstrating an acute focal hyperintense lesion with local cord swelling. The transverse plane allows localization of the lesion in respect to the cross-sectional extent

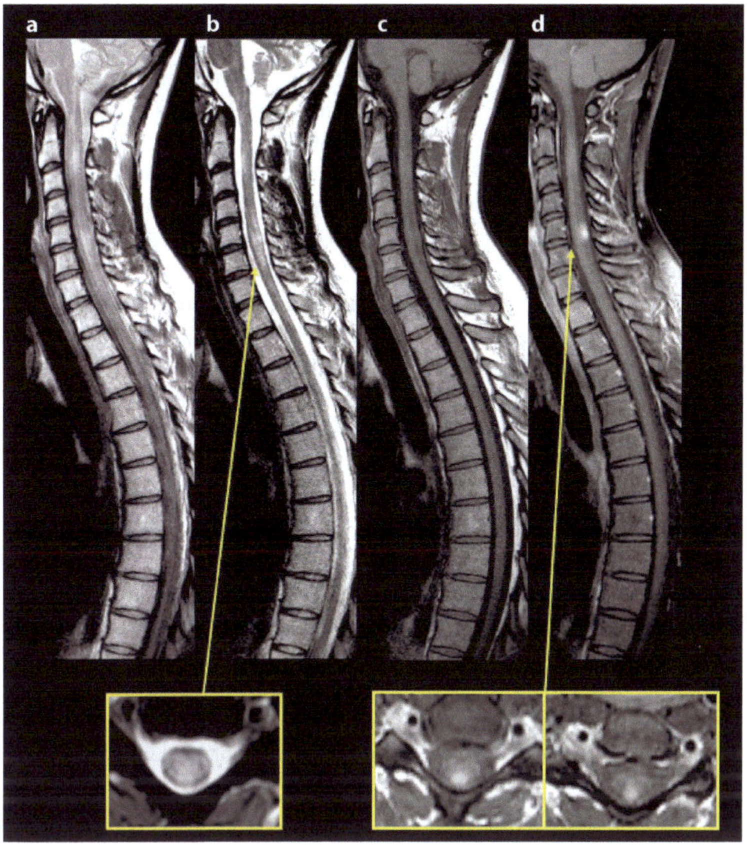

Fig. 7.8 Sagittal PD- (**a**), T2- (**b**), T1- (**c**), and T1-post–Gd-weighted (**d**) images of some chronic abnormality and an acute inflammatory cervical cord lesion. The acute focal lesion is noted with local swelling and pathological contrast enhancement on the sagittal T1-weighted image. The transverse images demonstrate the location of the lesion in the dorsal aspect of the cord

References

1. Adams RD, Kubik CS (1952) The morbid anatomy of the demyelinative diseases. Am J Med 12:510–546
2. Bot JCJ, Barkhof F, Polman C, Lycklama G, de Groot V, Bergers E, Adèr H, Castelijns JA (2004) Spinal cord abnormalities in recently diagnosed MS patients. Neurology 62:226–233
3. Gass A, Filippi M, Rodegher ME et al (1998) Characteristics of chronic MS lesions in the cerebrum, brainstem, spinal cord and optic nerve on T1-weighted MRI. Neurology 50:548–550
4. Kidd D, Thorpe JW, Thompson AJ, Kendall BE, Moseley IF, MacManus DG, McDonald WI, Miller DH (1993) Spinal cord MRI using multi-array coils and fast spin echo. II Findings in multiple sclerosis. Neurology 43:2632–2637
5. Lycklama G, Thompson A, Filippi M, Miller D, Polman C, Fazekas F, Barkghof F (2003) Spinal-cord MRI in multiple sclerosis. Lancet Neurol 2:555–562
6. Rovaris M, Viti B, Ciboddo G, Capra R, Filippi M (2000) Cervical cord magnetic resonance imaging findings in systemic immune-mediated diseases. J Neurol Sci 176:128–130
7. Simon JH (2000) The contribution of spinal cord MRI to the diagnosis and differential diagnosis of multiple sclerosis. J Neurol Sci (Suppl 1):S32–S35
8. Tartaglino LM, Friedman DP, Flanders AE, Lublin FD, Knobler RI, Liem M (1995) Multiple sclerosis in the spinal cord: MR appearance and correlation with clinical parameters. Radiology 195:725–732
9. Thielen KR, Miller GM (1996) Multiple sclerosis of the spinal cord: magnetic resonance appearance. J Comput Assist Tomogr 20:434–438
10. Thorpe JW, Kidd D, Kendall BE, Tofts PS, Barker GJ, Thompson AJ, MacManus DG, McDonald WI, Miller DH (1993) Spinal cord MRI using multi-array coils and fast spin echo. I Technical aspects and findings I healthy adults. Neurology 43:2625–2631

8 Diagnosis of Multiple Sclerosis

M.A. Sahraian, L. Kappos

8.1 Introduction. Revised McDonald Criteria

MS is a clinical diagnosis that depends on a detailed history, careful neurologic examination, and supportive paraclinical investigations. In fact, the diagnosis is based on the principle of dissemination in time and space of a disease compatible with MS in the absence of a better explanation. This principle was codified in 1983 by the Poser Committee, specifying that the diagnosis of clinically definite MS could be based on two attacks and clinical evidence of two lesions. For a clinical diagnosis, at least two clear episodes demonstrating involvement of two different parts of the CNS, lasting for 24 hours or more (relapse) and more than 30 days between the attacks are needed. According to Poser, MRI could fulfill the diagnostic criteria by showing another site of involvement in patients with two attacks and clinical evidence of one lesion (Poser et al. 1983). With expansion of knowledge on the predictive value of MRI in high-risk patients at their first clinical episode (O'Riordan et al. 1998), new diagnostic criteria for MS were proposed by an international panel chaired by Ian McDonald, which have increasingly found worldwide acceptance (McDonald et al. 2001). According to these criteria, the diagnosis of MS requires objective evidence of lesions disseminated in time and space, but MRI findings may contribute to the determination of these disseminations. Other supportive investigations include CSF and visually evoked potentials (VEPs).

For dissemination in space, the Barkhof-Tintore MRI criteria that require three out of the following four elements have been included in the McDonald criteria:

1. At least one Gd enhancing lesion or nine T2 hyperintense lesions
2. At least one infratentorial lesion
3. At least one juxtacortical lesion
4. At least three periventricular lesions

In the light of subsequent studies and criticism, the 2001 criteria were revised for a more rapid diagnosis, clarifying the use of spinal cord lesions and simplifying the diagnosis of primary progressive MS.

A constant feature in both the 2001 and the 2005 criteria is the use of the Barkhof-Tintore criteria for demonstrating dissemination in space. In the revised form dissemination in time can be demonstrated by:

- Detection of a Gd enhancing lesion at least 3 months after the onset of the initial clinical event, if not at the site corresponding to the initial event
- Detection of a new T2 lesion if it appears at any time, compared with a reference scan done at least 30 days after the onset of the initial clinical event

The reason for selecting the 30-day period is to exclude new T2 lesions occurring in the first few weeks after the onset of the first clinical episode, which would not be considered a new separate event.

The new revised criteria also differ in the extent to which a spinal cord lesion can assist with fulfillment of dissemination in space: In 2001, only one cord lesion could substitute for one brain lesion, whereas in 2005 any number of cord lesions can substitute for brain lesions. In addition, a cord lesion is also assigned the same status as an infratentorial lesion. Finally, another change to the original McDonald criteria has been proposed for diagnosis of primary progressive MS (Table 8.1). In primary progressive MS, the presence of CSF oligoclonal band is no longer required, though in their absence it is necessary to have at least two spinal cord lesions and either nine brain lesions or four to eight brain lesions plus abnormal VEPs (Polman et al. 2005).

It should be noted that even with wide utility of MRI in MS, diagnosis should remain based on clinical setting and judgment. The other important point is the exclusion of other possible etiologies that can mimic MS in clinical presentation or MRI findings (see Chap. 9).

The present chapter deals with diagnosis of MS, demonstrating several examples for demonstrating dissemination in time and space by MRI.

Table 8.1 The 2005 revisions to the McDonald Diagnostic Criteria for Multiple Sclerosis

Clinical presentation	Additional data needed for diagnosing MS
Two or more attacks[a]; objective clinical evidence of two or more lesions	None[b]
Two or more attacks[a]; objective clinical evidence of one lesion	Dissemination in space demonstrated by: MRI[c] *or* Two or more MRI-detected lesions consistent with MS plus positive CSF[d] *or* Await further clinical attack[a] implicating a different site
One attack[a]; objective clinical evidence of two or more lesions	Dissemination in time demonstrated by: MRI[e] *or* Second clinical attack[a]
One attack[a]; objective clinical evidence of one lesion (monosymptomatic presentation; clinically isolated syndrome)	Dissemination in space demonstrated by: MRI[c] *or* Two or more MRI-detected lesions consistent with MS plus positive CSF[d] *and* Dissemination in time demonstrated by: MRI[e] *or* Second clinical attack[a]
Insidious neurological progression suggestive of MS	One year of disease progression (retrospectively or prospectively determined) *and* Two of the following: positive brain MRI (nine T2 lesions or four or more T2 lesions with positive VEP)[f] Positive spinal cord MRI (two focal T2 lesions) Positive CSF[d]

If the criteria indicated are fulfilled and there is no better explanation for the clinical presentation, the diagnosis is MS; if suspicious, but criteria are not completely met, the diagnosis is "possible MS"; if another diagnosis arises during the evaluation that better explains the entire clinical presentation, then the diagnosis is "not MS"

[a] An *attack* is defined as an episode of neurological disturbance for which causative lesions are likely to be inflammatory and demyelinating in nature. There should be subjective report (back-up by objective findings) or objective observation that the event lasts for at least 24 h

[b] No additional tests are required; however, if tests (MRI, CSF) are undertaken and are negative, extreme caution needs to be taken before making a diagnosis of MS. Alternative diagnosis must be considered. There must be no better explanation for clinical picture and some objective evidence to support a diagnosis of MS

[c] MRI demonstration of space dissemination must fulfill the criteria derived from Barkhof and colleagues and Tintore and coworkers as presented in the text

[d] Positive CSF determined by oligoclonal bands detected by established methods (isoelectric focusing) different from any such bands in serum, or by an increased immunoglobulin G (IgG) index

[e] MRI demonstration of time dissemination must fulfill the criteria explained in the text

[f] Abnormal VEP of type seen in MS

8.2 Images

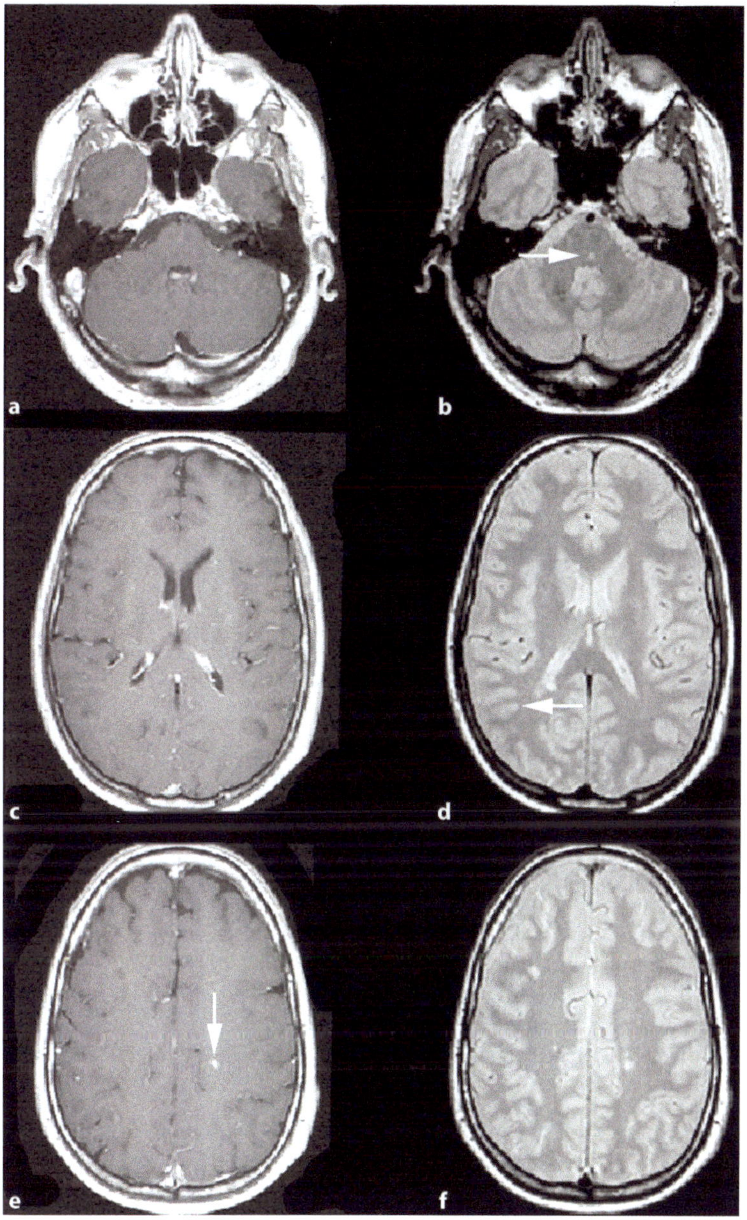

Fig. 8.1 Axial T1-weighted with contrast (**a,c,e**) and PD (**b,d,f**) images of a young woman who presented with paresthesia of the right arm. MRI was performed with the impression of a demyelinating disease. Does this MRI fulfill the criteria for dissemination in space? Note: Brain MRI demonstrates at least one enhancing lesion, one infratentorial, and one juxtacortical lesion (*arrows*), so this patient fulfills the criteria for dissemination in space

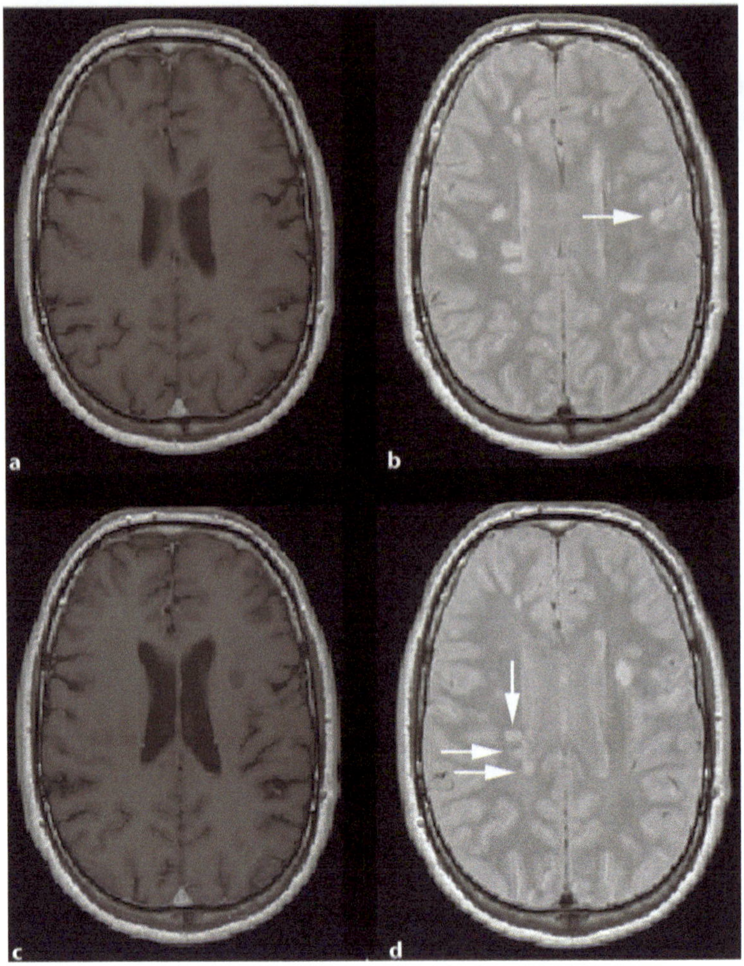

Fig. 8.2 Axial T1-weighted with contrast (**a**,**c**) and PD (**b**,**d**) images of a patient who presented with unilateral optic neuritis. Cranial MRI was performed with impression of MS. Does this MRI fulfill the criteria for dissemination in space? Note: This MRI shows at least one juxtacortical, three periventricular, and nine T2-weighted lesion (*arrows*). The criteria for dissemination in space are fulfilled

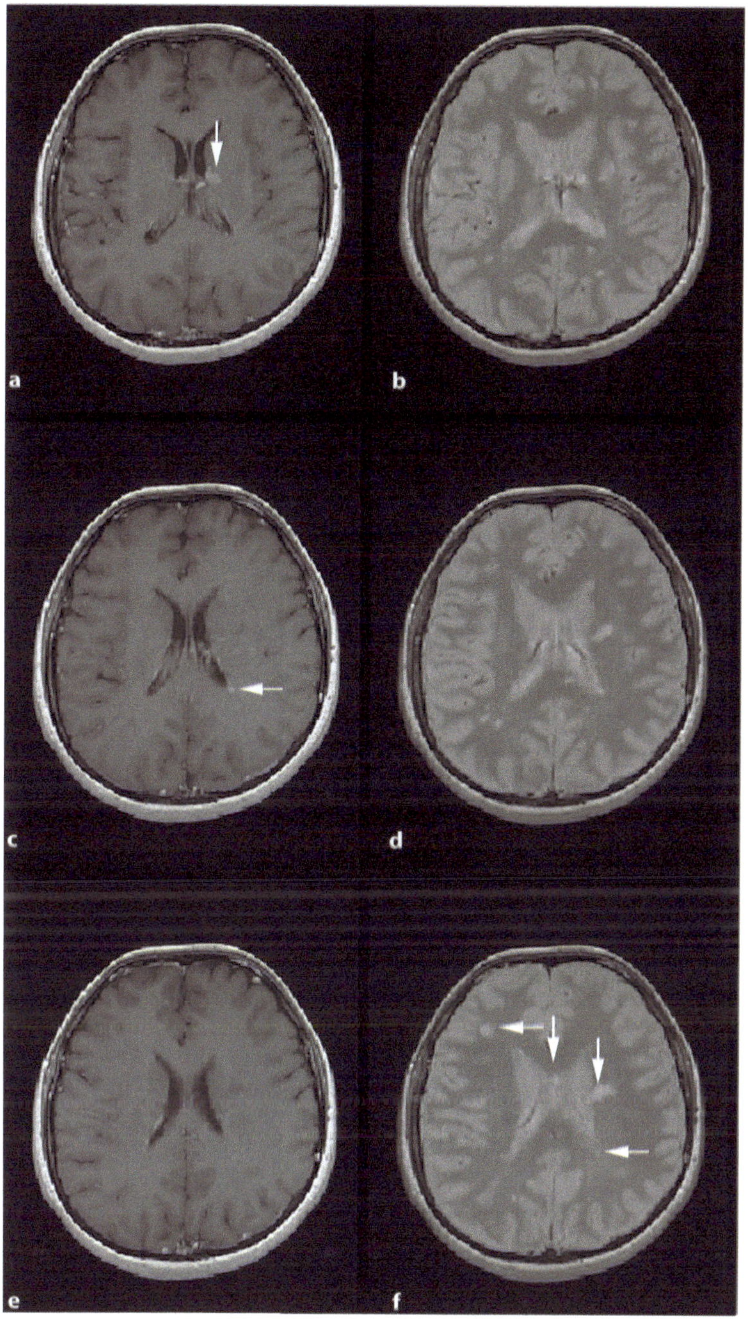

Fig. 8.3 Axial T1-weighted with contrast (**a,c,e**) and PD (**b,d,f**) images of a patient with paresthesia of the lower extremities and bilateral Babinski's signs. Does the brain MRI fulfill the criteria for dissemination in space? Note: This brain MRI demonstrates dissemination in space because the patient has at least one enhancing, one juxtacortical, and three periventricular lesions (*arrows*)

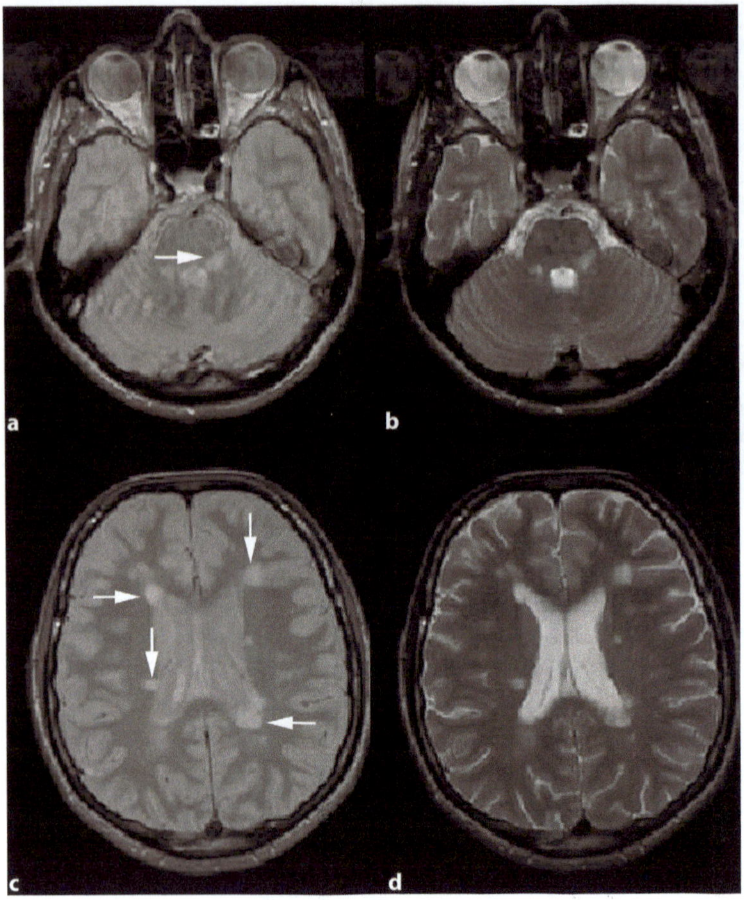

Fig. 8.4 Axial PD- (a,c) and T2-weighted (**b**,**d**) images of a patient suspected for MS show dissemination in space with at least one infratentorial, one juxtacortical, and three periventricular lesions (*arrows*)

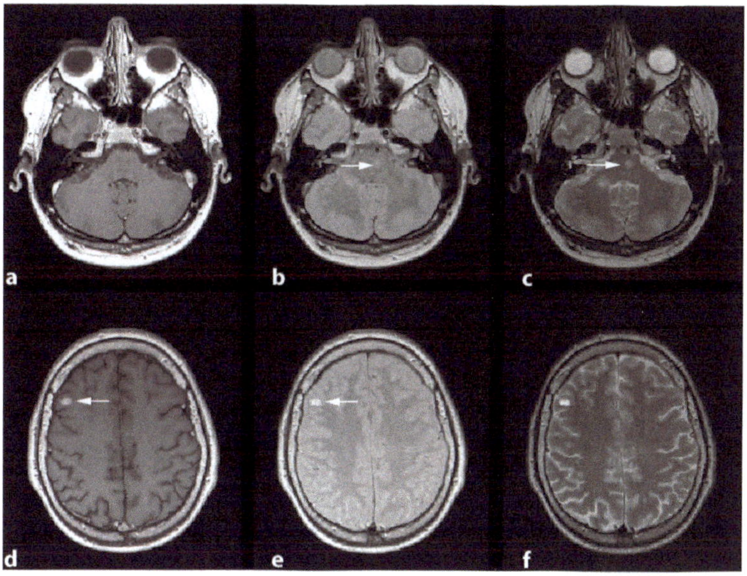

Fig. 8.5 Axial T1-weighted with contrast (**a**,**d**), PD- (**b**,**e**), and T2-weighted (**c**,**f**) images of a young patient who presented with ataxia and nystagmus. MRI was performed with the impression of a demyelinating disease. Does this MRI fulfill the criteria for dissemination in space? Note: This patient demonstrates an enhancing juxtacortical lesion and at least one infratentorial lesion that fulfill the criteria

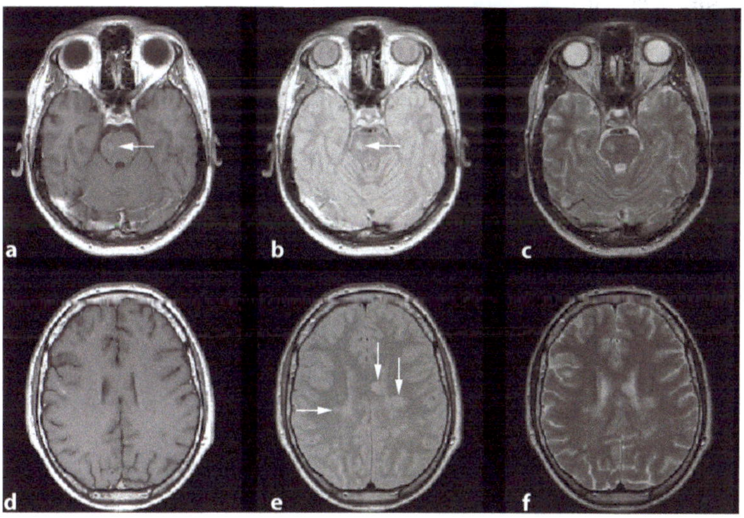

Fig. 8.6 Axial T1-weighted with contrast (**a**,**d**), PD- (**b**,**e**), and T2-weighted (**c**,**f**) images of a patient suspected for MS demonstrate dissemination in space, with an enhancing lesion of the pons, its corresponding T2 abnormality, and three periventricular lesions (*arrows*)

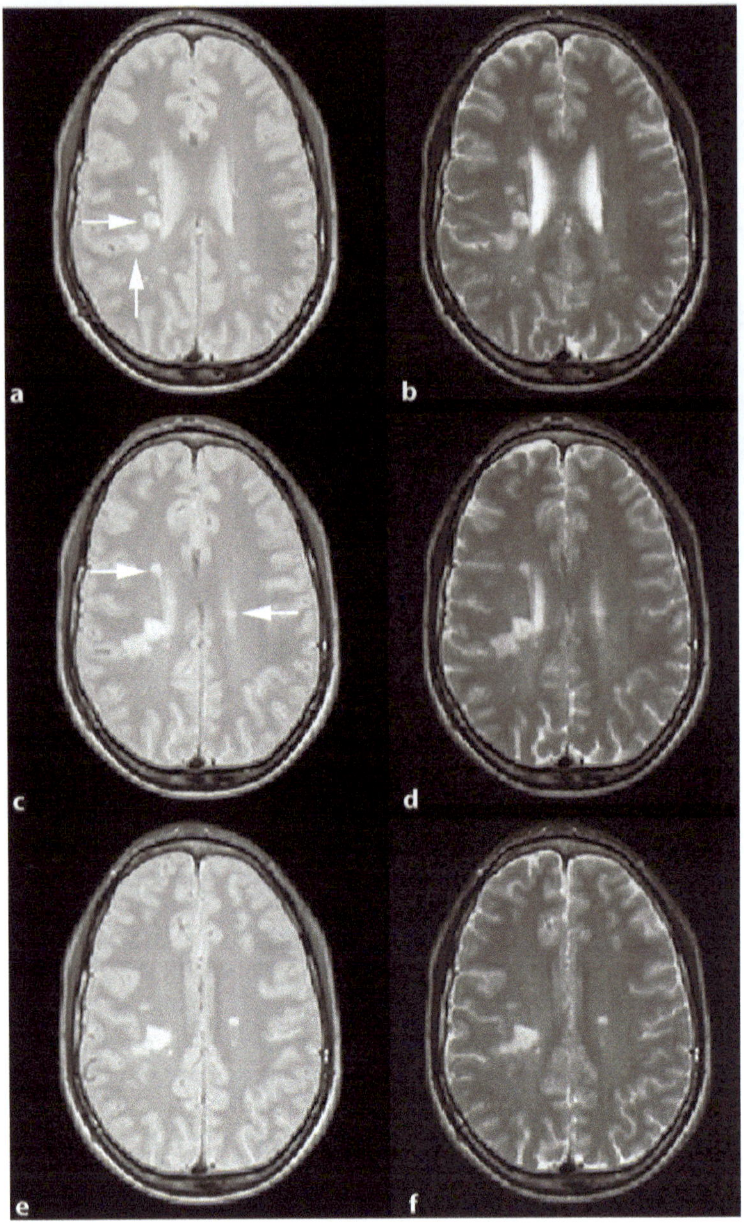

Fig. 8.7 Axial PD- (**a,c,e**) and T2-weighted (**b,d,f**) images of a patient who presented with left-side hypoesthesia demonstrate several hyperintense lesions compatible with a demyelinating disorder. The presence of at least one juxtacortical, three periventricular, and nine T2 lesions fulfill the criteria for dissemination in space (*arrows*)

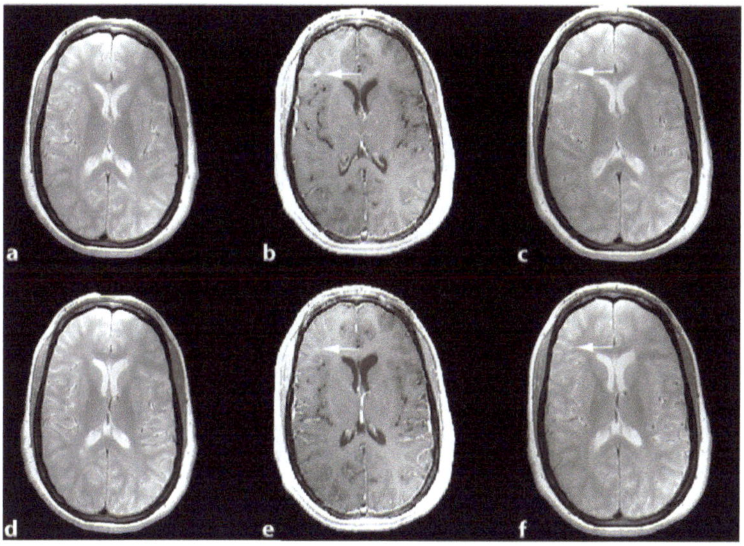

Fig. 8.8 Axial baseline (**a**,**d**) images of a patient who presented with unilateral optic neuritis and follow-up after 3 months (**b**,**c**,**e**,**f**) demonstrate a new enhancing lesion with its corresponding T2 abnormality (*arrows*). Note: This patient fulfills the criteria for dissemination in time with the new enhancing lesion after 3 months

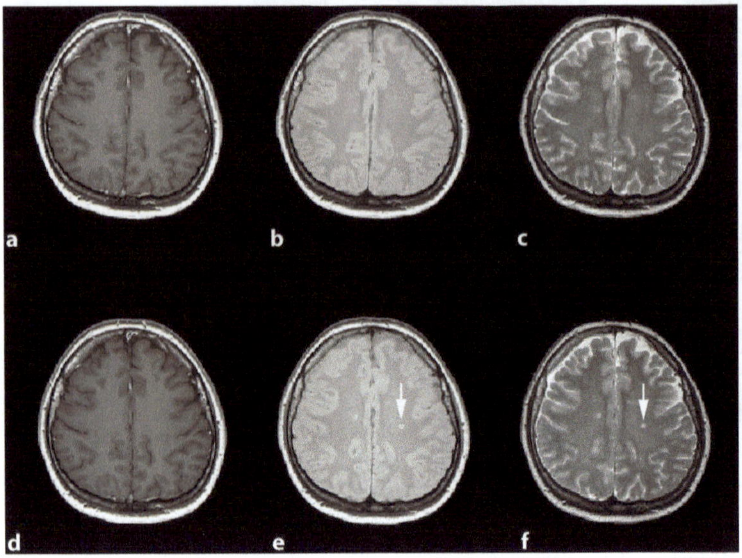

Fig. 8.9 Axial baseline (**a–c**) images of a young girl who presented with unilateral optic neuritis and their follow-up after 1 month (**d–f**) that demonstrate a new T2 lesion (*arrow*). Baseline MRI was performed 5 days after symptom appearance. Does follow up MRI fulfill the criteria for dissemination in time? Note: This patient does not fulfill the criteria for dissemination in time because this new T2 lesion may have developed during the first month after symptoms. Dissemination in time is demonstrated by the appearance of new T2 lesions on a reference scan done at any time but at least 30 days after onset of symptoms

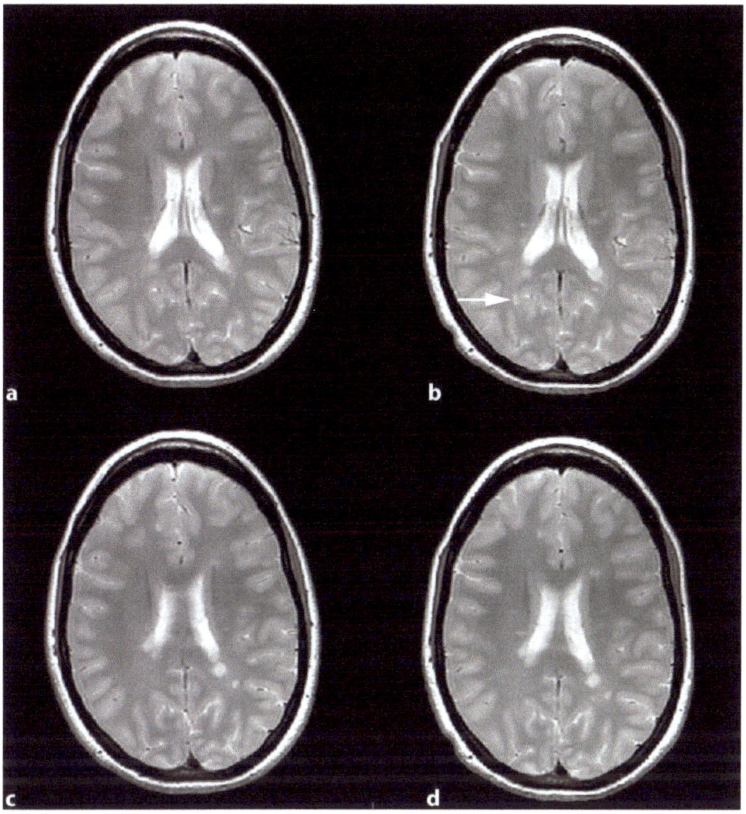

Fig. 8.10 Axial baseline (a,c) images of a patient who presented with paresthesia of the lower extremities and hyperreflexia. The follow-up images after 3 months (b,d) demonstrate a new T2-weighted lesion. Baseline MRI was performed 1 month after the onset of symptoms. Note: This patient fulfills the criteria for dissemination in time with a new T2-weighted abnormality after 3 months, as the reference scan has been performed 1 month after onset of symptoms

References

1. Barkhof F, Filippi M, Miller DH et al (1997) Comparison of MRI criteria at first presentation to predict conversion to clinically definite multiple sclerosis. Brain 120:2059–2069
2. Mc Donald WI, Compston A, Edan G et al (2001) Recommended diagnostic criteria for multiple sclerosis: guidelines from the International Panel on the Diagnosis of Multiple Sclerosis. Ann Neurol 50:121–127
3. O'Riordan JI, Thompson AJ, Kingsley DP et al (1998) The prognostic value of brain MRI in clinically isolated syndromes of the CNS: a 10-year follow-up. Brain 121:495–503
4. Polman C, Reingold SC, Edan G et al (2005) Diagnostic criteria for multiple sclerosis: 2005 revisions to the McDonald criteria. Ann Neurol 58:840–846
5. Poser CM, Paty DW, Scheinberg L et al (1983) New diagnostic criteria for multiple sclerosis: guidelines for research protocols. Ann Neurol 13:227–231

9 Differential Diagnosis of Multiple Sclerosis

J. Kira, S. Haller, J. Kesselring, M. A. Sahraian

9.1 Introduction

The signs and symptoms related to MS are diverse and white matter abnormalities on MRI are not specific. In a small number of patients with MS brain MRI may be normal and in others it may show diffuse, large or atypical lesions. As there is no paraclinical test that is pathognomonic for MS and many conditions can mimic this disease clinically or radiologically, the new Mc Donald's criteria still insist on the exclusion of alternative conditions for correct diagnosis of MS (Polman et al. 2005). In fact, diagnosis of MS is based on showing disease dissemination in space and time and on the exclusion of other diseases that may explain the neurological symptoms of the patients.

Many white matter diseases may mimic MS, with or without extension to the gray matter (Table 9.1), but in this chapter we focus on those disorders that pose diagnostic difficulties or are frequently reported in patients suspicious for MS. For each disease, we try to have some clinical overview and also to review MRI findings in order to facilitate differentiation from multiple sclerosis.

9.2 Systemic Immune-Mediated Diseases

Systemic immune-mediated diseases can affect the CNS. Several of these disorders can involve white matter and cause remitting-relapsing or progressive neurological deterioration. Isolated CNS involvement is infrequent, and usually there are evident systemic features leading to a correct diagnosis.

Several vasculitic disorders may involve the brain like systemic lupus erythematosus (SLE), Wegener's granulomatosis, Behçet's syndrome, and periarteritis nodosa, but we shall review SLE and Behçet's disease as the most important ones. Sarcoidosis is also discussed under this heading, although its precise etiology is not known.

9.2.1 Systemic Lupus Erythematosus

Neurologic manifestations usually occur in the setting of known lupus, but about 3% of the patients present with CNS involvement. Clinical signs of CNS involvement are highly diverse and often have major prognostic consequences. The most common neurological manifestations are neuropsychiatric syndromes, seizure, aseptic meningitis, vascular events, movement disorders, transverse myelitis, and optic nerve involvement (Jennekens and Kater 2002).

MRI changes are nonspecific and may reveal small or large cerebral infarcts and vessel irregularities. Small vessels angiopathy due to lupus may appear as small punctual lesions of increased signal intensity, located mainly in the periventricular and subcortical white and gray matter. These multiple periventricular and subcortical lesions may mimic MS classic appearance. Gd enhancement is less common than in

MS, and T1 black holes are rarely seen (Fig. 9.1) (Jennekens et al. 2004).

9.2.2 Behçet's Disease

Behçet's disease is another systemic vasculitis that presents with recurrent oral and genital ulcers and intraocular inflammation. Although neurological involvement is less frequent than with other major presentations, it is important because it produces severe disability and is associated with a bad prognosis. Involvement of CNS usually presents after systemic manifestations, but in the minority of patients (about 3%), neurologic findings clearly antedated other common signs of illness (Akman-Demir et al. 1999). Neurological manifestations include focal meningoencephalitis, cerebrovascular syndromes, seizures, cranial neuropathies, myelopathy and encephalopathy. The disease may follow a relapsing-remitting course. MRI shows multiple patchy foci of increased signal intensity on T2-weighted images, which may be hypointense on T1-weighted images. The lesions enhance during the acute phase, and enhancement resolves rapidly after steroid treatment. The most common sites of involvement are the mesodiencephalic junction, cerebral peduncles, pons, midbrain, and spinal cord. Basal ganglia, internal capsules, and optic nerves may also be involved. In hemispheric lesions there is no predilection for the periventricular regions in comparison with MS plaques (Borhani Haghighi et al. 2005). Brainstem lesions without any cerebral white matter changes may be seen in Behçet's disease but it is quite unusual in MS (Figs. 9.3, 9.4).

9.2.3 Sarcoidosis

Sarcoidosis is a multisystem granulomatous disease with unknown etiology. The lungs are affected most frequently, but eyes, nervous system, heart, kidneys, and bones may also be affected. Involvement of the nervous system is referred to as neurosarcoidosis and occurs in 5% of the patients. Neurosarcoidosis is most commonly seen during the fourth and fifth decades of life, but the disease can affect children and the elderly as well. Both central and peripheral nervous system may be affected. Involvement of different parts of the CNS such as cranial nerves, pituitary gland, and hypothalamus may result in diverse signs and symptoms like facial palsy, optic neuritis, polyuria, polydipsia, and other symptoms of hormonal disturbances. Involvement of brain parenchyma and the overlying meninges results in headache, seizure, or impaired consciousness. Brain MRI reveals prominent meningeal enhancement, hypothalamic involvement, hydrocephalus, and multifocal white matter lesions. Acute lesions may enhance, which regress with steroid therapy. Although MRI may have the same appearance as is usually found in MS, meningeal enhancement, presence of hydrocephalus and punctiform parenchymal enhancement help in differentiation (Lexa and Grossman 1994). Diagnostic workup includes sedimentation rate, serum level of converting enzyme, and computed tomography of the chest (Figs. 9.5, 9.6, 9.7).

9.3 Noninflammatory Vascular Syndromes

9.3.1 Binswanger's Disease

Ischemia of the deep central white matter is believed to be the basis of Binswanger's disease. The patients present with cognitive impairment and behavioral abnormalities. Psuedobulbar palsy, pyramidal tract signs, and gait abnormalities are common neurological findings. Some of the patients may develop psychomotor slowing and abulia. Brain MRI demonstrates extensive white matter changes as they appear in advanced MS.

The lesions are irregular, often slit-like, sparing the periventricular region and extending into the corona radiata. U-fibers are usually spared compared to multiple sclerosis.

The age of the patient at onset of clinical presentation and sparing of U-fibers on MRI help to differentiate Binswanger's disease from MS (Figs. 9.8, 9.9, 9.10) (Loeb 2000).

9.3.2 Cerebral Autosomal Dominant Arteriopathy with Subcortical Infarct and Leukoencephalopathy (CADASIL)

CADASIL results from mutation in the *notch 3* gene on chromosome 19 and is characterized by a widespread microangiopathy affecting small diameter arterioles. Neurological manifestations of CADASIL include relapsing-multifocal neurological deficits similar to those of MS. Brain MRI shows abnormalities in cerebral white matter, deep gray structures, and external capsule.

The MRI shows special involvement of the external capsule and temporal poles, which helps in diagnosis. Characteristic clinical features, skin biopsy, and genetic testing in suspected cases result in diagnosis (Figs. 9.11, 9.12).

9.3.3 Mitochondrial Encephalopathies

Mitochondrial cytopathies are a heterogeneous group of clinical entities that may present with stepwise or progressive neurological deterioration. The description of all genetic abnormalities and clinical syndromes of mitochondrial diseases is beyond the scale of this chapter but among this group, MELAS (mitochondrial encephalopathy epilepsy lactic acidosis and stroke) should be considered in the differential diagnosis of MS.

Clinically, MELAS presents with one or a mixture of the following manifestations: epileptic seizures, cognitive impairment, exercise intolerance, limb weakness, and stroke-like episodes, the latter giving rise to both reversible and permanent neurological deficits.

Hemiparesis, hemianopsia or cortical blindness are common manifestations. CT scan may show the presence of calcium deposits in the globus pallidus and caudate nucleus. MRI shows more cortical involvement than the underlying white matter. Cortical enhancement may be seen. The lesions are large, confluent, single or multiple, and usually asymmetrical.

The occipital and posterior areas are preferentially involved. In follow-up studies, MRI may show migrating infarctions that leave their traces in progressive atrophy with enlargement of the ventricles (Rosen et al. 1990). Calcium deposits may help in differentiation (Figs. 9.13, 9.14).

It should be noted that other mitochondrial cytopathies like myoclonic epilepsy associated with ragged red fibers (MERRF) can involve the CNS and cause progressive neurologic diseases.

9.4 Other Demyelinating Diseases

9.4.1 Acute Disseminated Encephalomyelitis (ADEM)

ADEM is an immune-mediated response to a preceding viral infection or vaccination. It predominantly affects children and is usually monophasic (Tenembaum et al. 2002).

The most common trigger is an unspecific upper respiratory tract infection, but many different viruses and bacterial infections have been reported to be the preceding event.

The neurological symptoms vary, depending on the size and location of the demyelinating lesions. The disease commonly presents with nonspecific symptoms including headache, vomitting, fever, drowsiness, and lethargy. Focal brainstem and/or hemispheric signs, transverse myelitis, cranial neuropathies, and cerebellar ataxia are the main neurological manifestations (Hynson et al. 2001; Tenembaum et al. 2002; Murthy et al. 2002).

Brain MRI demonstrates multifocal, commonly symmetrical lesions that may involve supra- and infratentorial regions. The lesions tend to have poorly defined borders and uniformly enhance during the acute phase (Gasperini 2001).

Relative absence of Dawson's fingers, periventricular lesions, and detection of the lesions at the same age may help in differentiating from MS. Lesions in ADEM typically involve basal ganglia and thalamus, a feature that is not common in MS. Moreover, many lesions resolve in serial MRI of ADEM, but in MS, some new lesions develop over time.

CSF findings are variable and range from unremarkable results to lymphatic pleocytosis and increase in protein. The spinal fluid usually contains no oligoclonal band, but its presence does not exclude the disease (Megni et al. 2005).

In summary, the following features help in differentiation ADEM from MS:

1. ADEM is more common in children, whereas MS is more common in adults. Most series of ADEM have failed to show sex predominance. By contrast, females are more predisposed to develop MS.
2. Most of the patients (50–75%) with ADEM have a history of a precipitating infection. Although infections may precipitate MS relapse, the association with infection is less pronounced.
3. ADEM patients commonly have headache, vomitting, and encephalopathy. These symptoms are uncommon in MS. Polysymptomatic presentation is much more common in ADEM than in MS.
4. Interathecal synthesis of oligoclonal bands is more common in MS than in ADEM.
5. Periventricular, corpus callosum, and white matter lesions are more common in MS, whereas basal ganglia and thalamus are more involved in ADEM.
6. The original lesions in ADEM resolve completely or partially over time, whereas in MS appearance of new lesions is anticipated (Figs. 9.15, 9.16) (Dale and Branson 2004).

9.4.2 Neuromyelitis Optica (NMO)

Devic's disease or neuromyelitis optica is an idiopathic inflammatory, demyelinating disease of the CNS characterized by sequential or synchronous attacks of optic neuritis and severe myelitis. Transverse myelitis is commonly complete, and optic neuritis may be bilateral. Recently, a serum autoantibody marker of neuromyelitis optica (NMO-5G6) has been identified, which provides a quantitative measure to differentiate NMO from MS.

MRI of the spinal cord demonstrates lesions typically extending contiguously over three or more vertebral segments on sagittal T2-weighted images. Lesions are usually located in the cord center and enhance with Gd, sometimes for several months (Figs. 9.17, 9.18) (Wingerchuk 2007).

9.4.3 Central Pontine Myelinolysis (CPM)

Central pontine myelinolysis is a demyelinating disease of the pons rarely associated with demyelination of the limbic system and subthalamic structures. The exact etiology and pathogenesis is not clear, but almost all cases of CPM relate to severe diseases. Chronic alcoholism is one of the most common underlying conditions (Lampl and Yazdi 2002). The correlation between CPM and hyponatremia was described for the first time in 1962. A number of cases have also been reported in the absence of hyponatremia; however, a rapid change in serum sodium level may play a more important role in the development of CPM than hyponatremia itself (Norenberg et al. 1982). The clinical picture is variable and includes psychiatric symptoms, disturbances of consciousness, impaired function of cranial nerves, and spastic paraparesis. Extreme cases may develop locked-in syndrome. MRI is the imaging modality of choice. Typically, T2-weighted MRI images demonstrate hyperintensity in the pons and in areas where demyelination has occurred (Fig. 9.20).

9.5 Infectious Diseases

9.5.1 Progressive Multifocal Leukoencephalopathy (PML)

Progressive multifocal leukoencephalopathy is a demyelinating disease of the CNS that is encountered most frequently in the setting of immune deficiency. The disease is caused by the human polyoma JC virus, a common and widespread infection in humans (Koralnik 2004). PML has also rarely been reported in subjects with no underlying disease, as a primary condition (Isella et al. 2005). Overall, HIV/AIDS has been estimated to be the underlying cause of immunosuppression in 55 to more than 85% of all current cases of PML (Major 1992). Seroepidemiological studies indicate that the JC virus has a worldwide distribution occurring generally at an early age (<20 years) (Berger and Houff 2004). As many as 80–90% of some populations have been exposed to this virus (Thumher et al. 1997). Following infection, the virus becomes latent in some tissues. Impairment of the immune system causes reactivation of the latent virus. Oligodendrocytes support the lytic cycle of JC virus infection, resulting in demyelination (Berger and Houff 2004). Clinical presentation is heterogeneous and shows no peculiarity with respect to the underlying disorders. The common clinical presentations include weakness, neuro-ophtalmologic disturbances such as homonymous hemianopsia or quadrantanopsia, and cognitive abnormalities. Sensory disturbances, seizures, headache, and vertigo are less frequent (Thumher et al. 1997).

Diagnosis depends on the clinical manifestations, MRI findings, and CSF examination. Biopsy supports the diagnosis in very doubtful cases.

PML has to be differentiated from other multifocal white matter disorders like MS.

MRI is the most sensitive tool for screening suspected patients for PML as it has the potential of detecting lesions at an early stage, possibly before they are clinically detectable.

The lesions appear as single or multiple high signal areas in T2-weighted images with variable shape and size. Typical PML lesions are diffuse, mainly subcortical, and located almost exclusively in white matter, although occasional extensions to gray matter and U-fibre involvement have been seen. The borders of the lesions are ill defined and irregular in shape. Typically there is no mass effect even in the large lesions, but they may slightly abut cerebral cortex. On T1-weighted sequences, lesions are slightly hypointense at onset, with signal intensity decreasing over time along the affected area. The lesions do not typically enhance, but some scant peripheral enhancement has been reported especially in HIV populations under treatment.

In follow-up images, PML lesions are usually progressive, and rapid involvement of other areas can be detected within 1 or 2 months. There is no reversion of signal intensity in T1-weighted lesions, and focal atrophy is usually not seen (Figs. 9.21, 9.22) (Yousry et al. 2006).

9.5.2 Human T-Cell Leukemia Virus 1 (HTLV1) Infection

Neurological manifestations of infection with HTLV1 do not mimic the typical relapsing-remitting MS but may be indistinguishable from the progressive form. The clinical manifestations are presence of thoracic myelopathy with bladder and bowel dysfunction and mild sensory disturbances (Ijichi and Osame 1995).

Spinal MRI reveals atrophy of the thoracic cord with or without abnormal increased signal and faint Gd enhancement.

Brain MRI may show scattered white matter lesions. Some cases have been reported with white matter lesions on brain MRI, indistinguishable from MS. CSF examination demonstrates oligoclonal band and a high local synthesis of HTLV1 antibodies (Douen et al. 1997)

9.5.3 Lyme Disease

The disease is caused by the tick-borne spirochete *Borrelia burgdorferi*. The neurological manifestations include meningitis, encephalitis, cranial neuritis, motor and sensory radicular neuritis, chorea, and myelitis.

MRI may reveal focal areas of high signal intensity on T2-weighted images with different patterns that may look very similarly to MS. It should be noted that not all cases with CNS symptoms have positive MRI findings, but because of the lesion pattern in MRI they should be considered as differential diagnosis for MS. Striking Gd enhancement of the meninges may help in differentiating Lyme disease from MS (Fig. 9.23).

9.6 Metabolic Diseases

9.6.1 Leukodystrophies

The leukodystrophies are familial disorders with onset usually in infancy or childhood. Adult forms of leukodystrophies may mimic progressive MS. Neurological manifestations include prominent cognitive decline, optic atrophy, nystagmus, spastic weakness, gait disturbances, and urinary dysfunction. Adrenoleukodystrophy may present during adulthood with behavioral abnormalities, pyramidal tract symptoms, slowly progressive myelopathy, and sometimes adrenal insufficiency. Brain MRI shows cerebral demyelination starting in the frontal white matter and spreading to the occipital white matter over time. Metachromatic leukodystrophy is the most common form of leukodystrophies and is inherited as autosomal recessive trait. The disease can begin at any age but usually starts between 1 and 3 years of age. Neurologic manifestations are cognitive decline, optic atrophy, nystagmus, spastic weakness, gait disturbance, urinary dysfunction, and peripheral neuropathy. Cranial MRI shows diffuse and symmetric abnormality of cerebral white matter (Trojano and Paolicelli 2001).

In summary, leukodystrophies present with diffuse, more or less symmetrical abnormalities. Involvement of the brainstem and cerebellum occur frequently. Selective symmetrical involvement of white matter tracts or nuclei suggests a metabolic rather than an acquired cause (Barkhof and Scheltens 2001).

White matter lesions tend to be non-enhancing, bilateral and symmetrical, which are important features to differentiate the disease from MS (Figs. 9.24, 9.25) (exception: adrenoleukodystrophy where lesions typically show peripheral enhancement).

9.7 Normal Aging Phenomenon

Multifocal areas of high signal intensity in T2-weighted images have been reported in more than 30% of healthy individuals over the age of 60 years. These hyperintensities can be located in the periventricular or deep white matter. Punctuate hyperintensities tend to be small and multiple. Large, confluent lesions with irregular border have also been reported. Arteriosclerosis and chronic ischemia have been discussed in the pathophysiology of such hyperintensities on T2-weighted images.

These nonspecific, age-related changes are not a problem in the differential diagnosis of most patients with MS who present before the age of 50 years. Small areas of extension and little posterior fossa involvement can help in differentiating such a phenomenon from patients with MS.

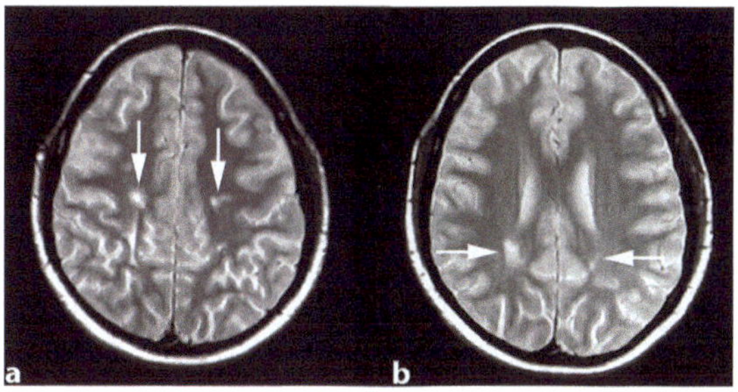

Fig. 9.1 Axial T2-weighted images of a patient with lupus demonstrate several hyperintense lesions of the white matter with different sizes (*arrows*). Note: Lupus may involve cerebral white and gray matter. Lesions may be small or large and may mimic MS lesions. Involvement of other organs, clinical presentations, and application of laboratory tests for lupus help to differentiate these two diseases

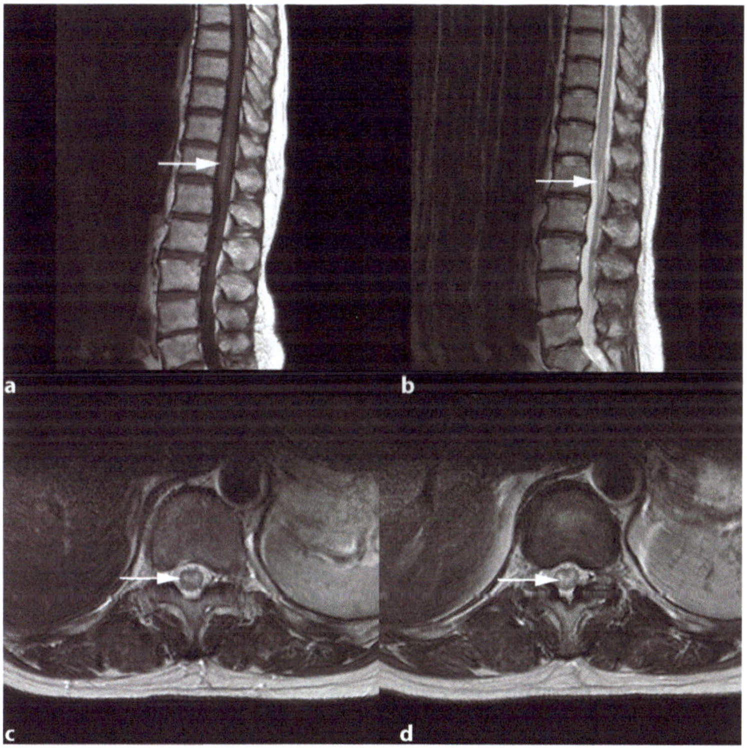

Fig. 9.2 Sagittal T1-weighted with contrast (**a**) and T2-weighted (**b**) images of a patient with antiphospholipid antibodies demonstrate involvement of the conus medullaris (*arrows*). T2 axial images are demonstrated in **c** and **d**. Note: Collagen vascular diseases—especially lupus and antiphospholipid syndrome—may involve the spinal cord and cause acute myelitis. These two diseases can even induce recurrent myelitis, but cord involvement usually occurs in patients with additional other systemic signs and symptoms

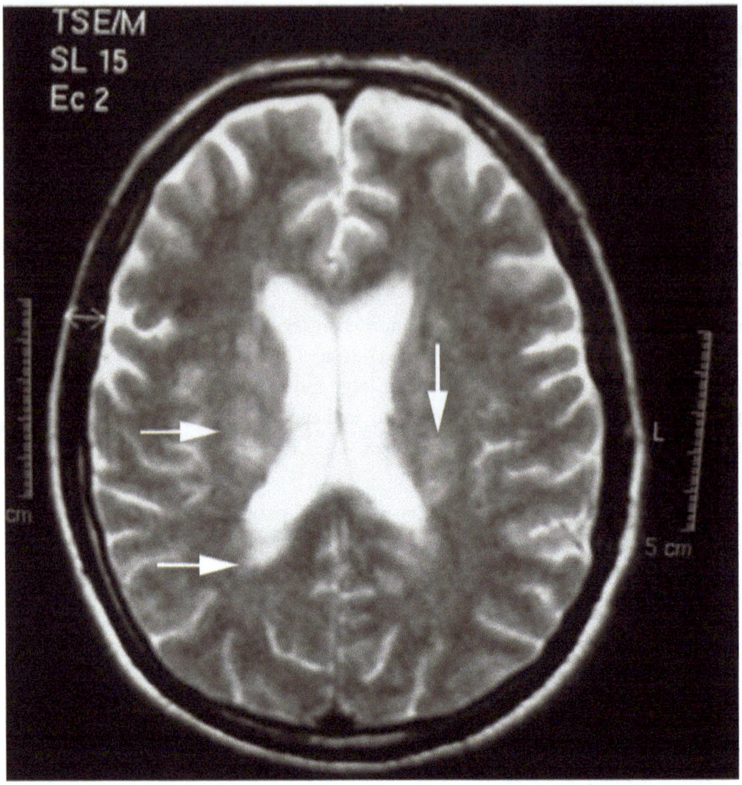

Fig. 9.3 Axial T2-weighted image of a patient with Behçet's disease demonstrate several ill-defined hyperintense lesions around the lateral ventricles (*arrows*). Note: The most common MRI abnormalities seen in Behçet's disease are multifocal cerebral white and gray matter lesions. Periventricular involvement is not common and the lesions tend to involve posterior fossa

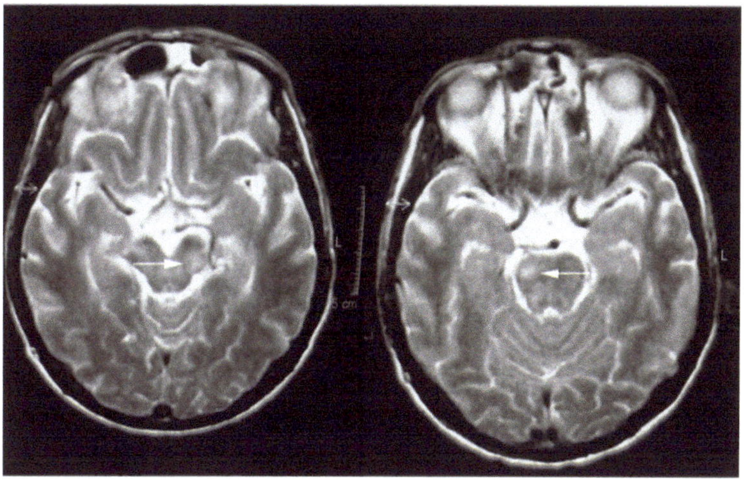

Fig. 9.4 Axial T2-weighted selected images of a patient with Behçet's disease demonstrate pontine involvements (*arrows*). Note: A predilection has been noted for mesodiencephalic junction. Involvement of the brainstem with relative sparing of supratentorial structures should raise the question of Behçet's disease

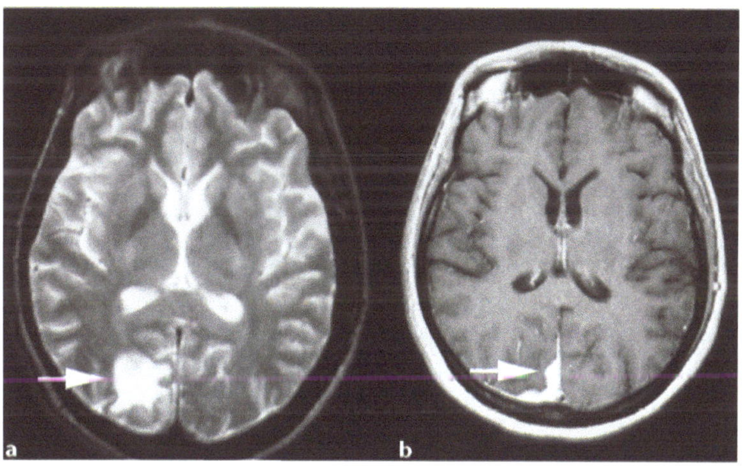

Fig. 9.5 Axial T2-weighted (**a**) and T1-weighted with contrast (**b**) image of a patient with sarcoidosis demonstrate involvement of right occipital lobe. The lesion is hypo- to isointense on the T2-weighted image, with edema around it. The lesion has been enhanced after contrast injection as well as the meninges around it. Note: Sarcoidosis may involve both white and gray matter separately or at the same time. The lesions may mimic MS lesions and enhance homogeneously in the acute phase. Most of the patients have involvement of the spinal cord and other organs, especially the lungs

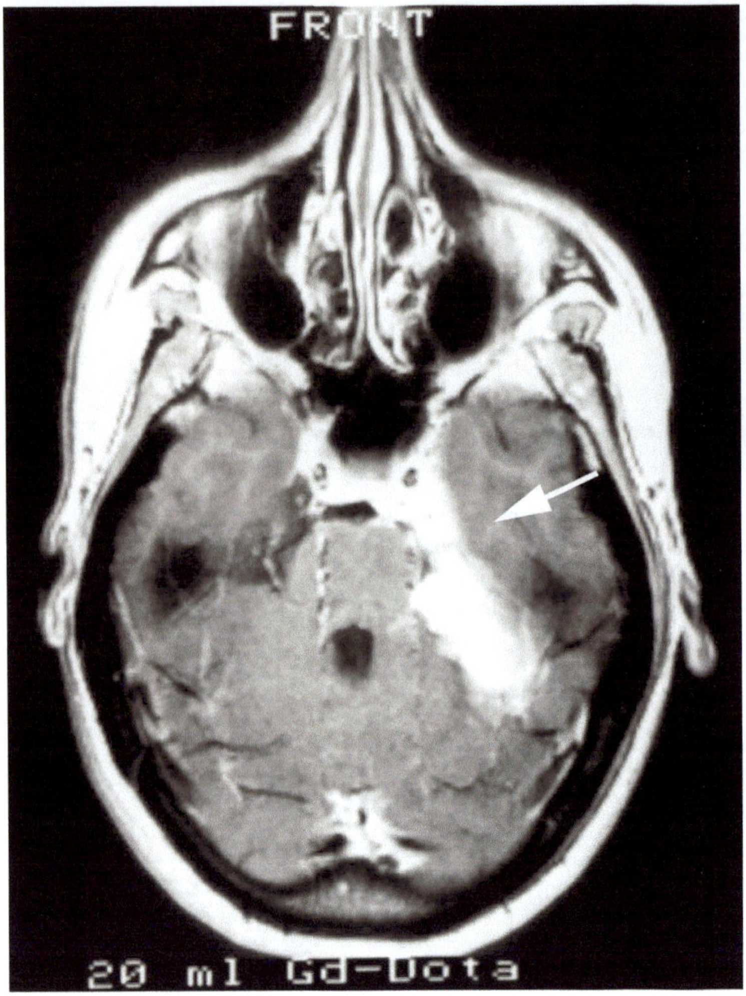

Fig. 9.6 Axial T1-weighted image with contrast of a patient with sarcoidosis demonstrate an enhancing lesion in the left pontocerebellar angle, with severe meningeal enhancement and involvement of the cavernous sinus (*arrow*)

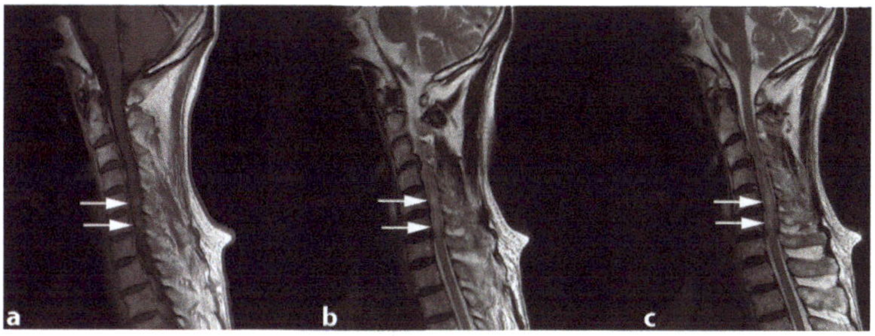

Fig. 9.7 Sagittal T1-weighted with contrast (**a**) and T2-weighted (**b**,**c**) images of a patient with sarcoidosis demonstrate intramedullary signal abnormalities in the cervical cord. The lesion has enhanced after contrast injection. Note: Spinal cord involvement in sarcoidosis may mimic MS both in clinical presentation and imaging, but the lesions may extend longer than do typical MS lesions

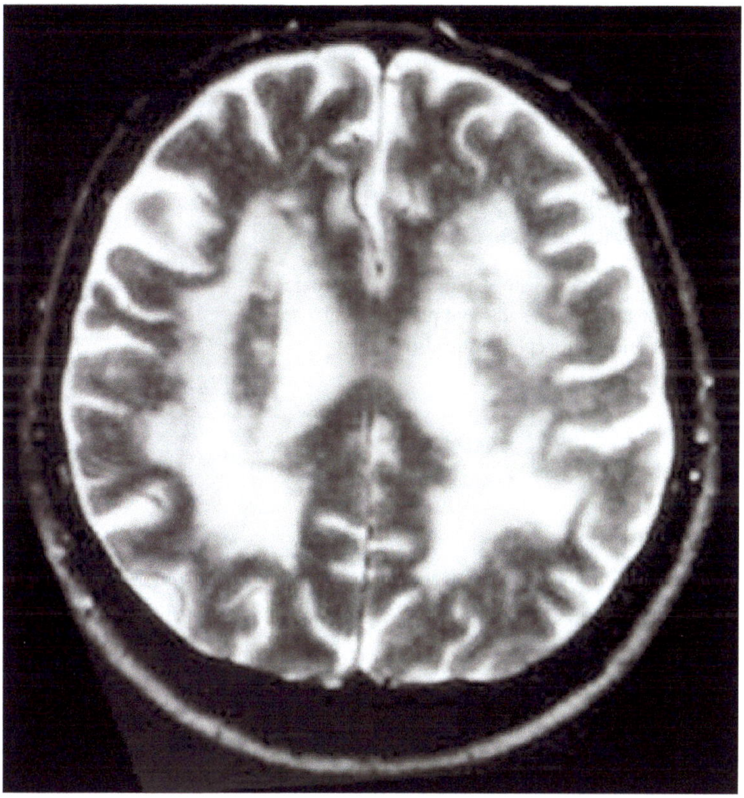

Fig. 9.8 Axial T2-weighted images of a patient with Binswanger's disease demonstrate disease involvement of white matter bilaterally. Note: Diffuse hyperintense changes in both hemispheres with relative sparing of U-fibers and the area adjacent to the ventricles are typical MRI features of Binswanger's disease

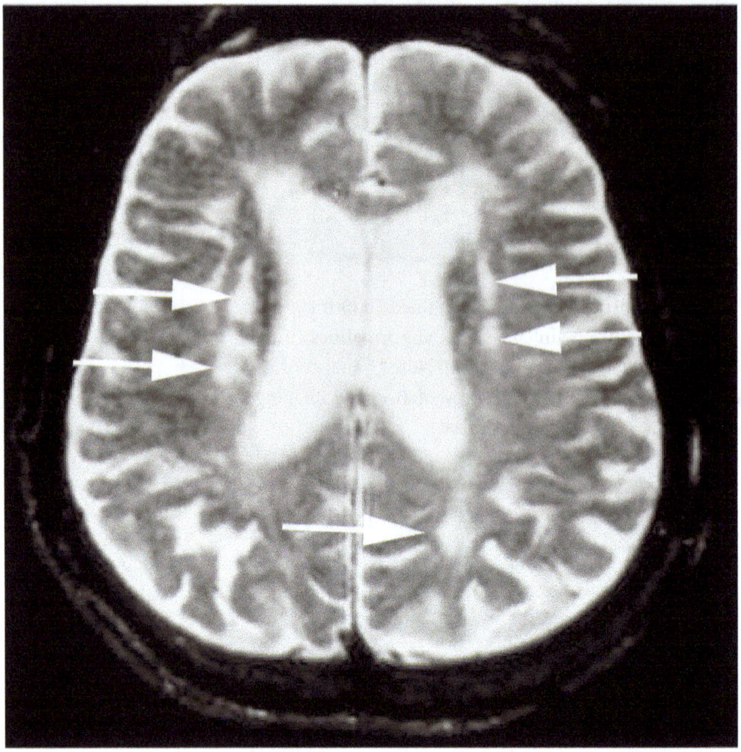

Fig. 9.9 Axial T2-weighted image of a patient with vascular dementia demonstrate multiple focal hyperintense lesions sparing the adjacent periventricular space (*arrows*). Diffuse white matter changes and hydrocephalus are also present

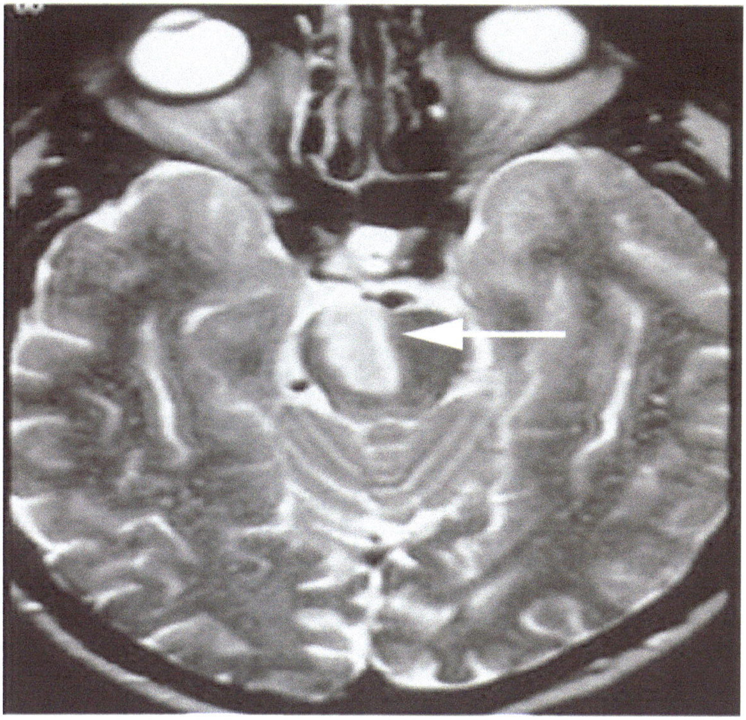

Fig. 9.10 Axial T2-weighted image of a patient with pontine infarction. Note: Brainstem infarctions especially may mimic MS lesions if they occur in young adults

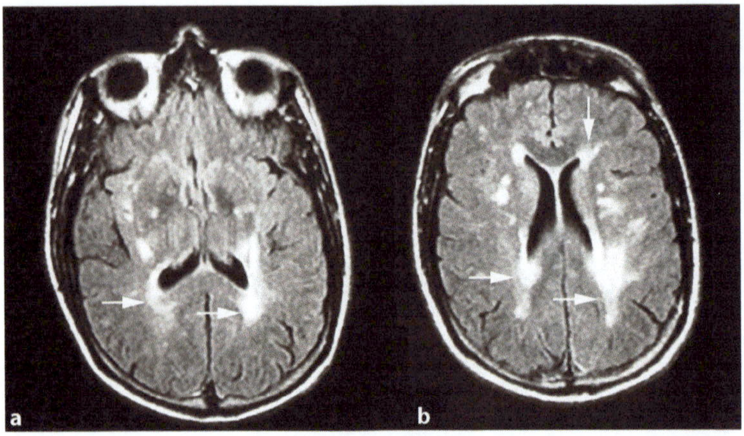

Fig. 9.11 Axial FLAIR selected images of a patient with CADASIL demonstrate multiple hyperintense discrete and confluent lesions in different parts of the cerebral hemisphere. Note: MRI findings in CADASIL are variable and range from focal small periventricular or juxtacortical hyperintensities on T2-weighted images to diffuse confluent lesions, involving white matter, especially temporobasal and sometimes basal ganglia or brainstem. Clinical evaluation and genetic testing help in differentiating from MS

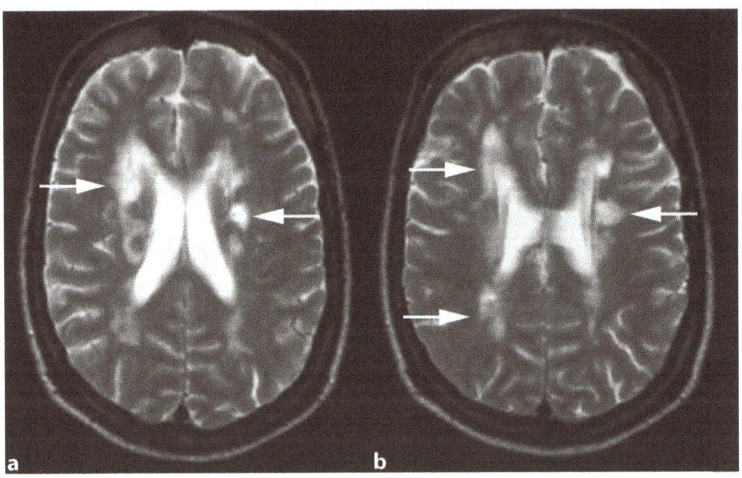

Fig. 9.12 Axial T2-weighted images of a patient with CADASIL demonstrate several hyperintense lesions around the lateral ventricle. Note: MRI appearance of CADASIL may mimic classic MS MRI features, but lack of callosal lesions and Dawson's fingers help in differentiation

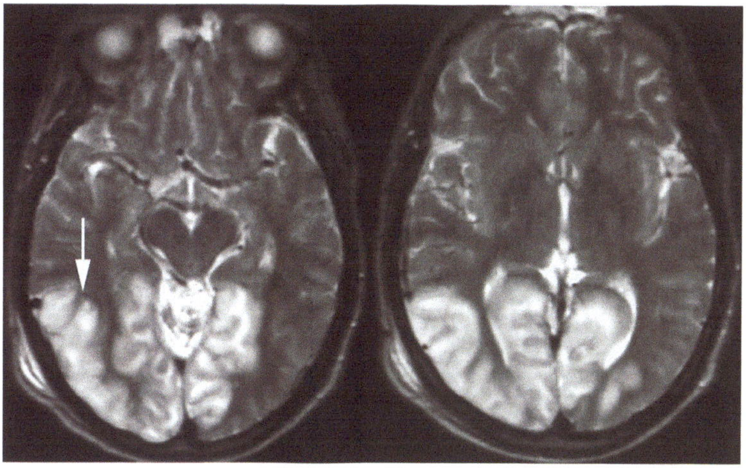

Fig. 9.13 Axial T2-weighted images of a patient with MELAS demonstrate severe involvement of the cerebral cortex and underlying white matter. MELAS tends to involve posterior part of the brain. Cortical involvement is more prominent than it is in MS

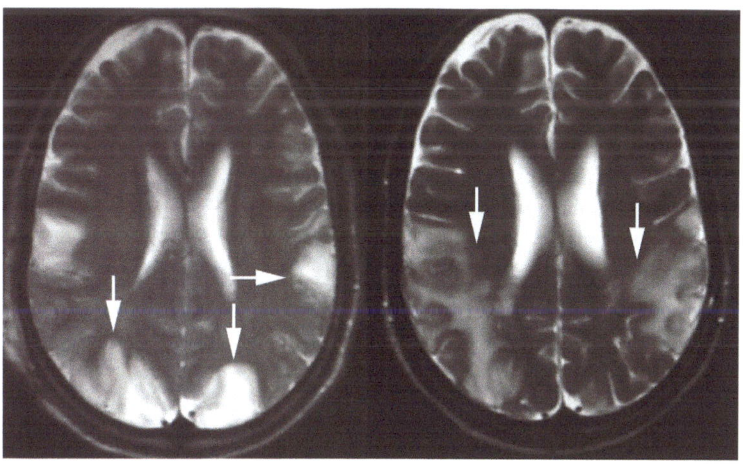

Fig. 9.14 Axial T2-weighted images of a patient with MELAS demonstrate involvement of both parieto-occipital regions at baseline (Fig. 9.13). The follow-up image after 3 months demonstrates partial resolution of previous lesions and involvement of new areas

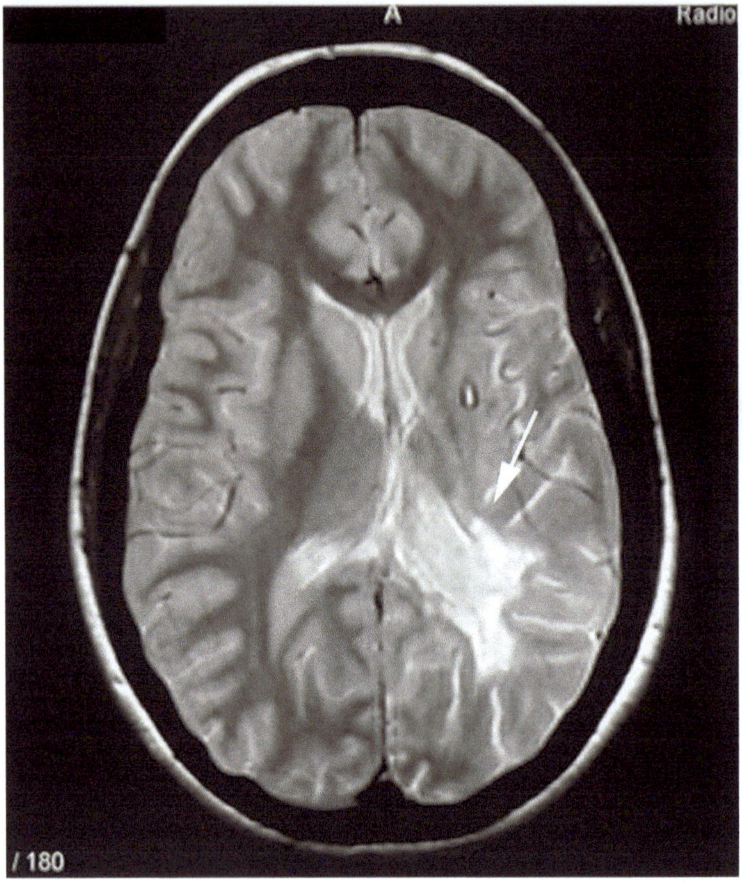

Fig. 9.15 Axial PD image of a patient with ADEM demonstrates a hyperintense lesion around the ventricle and deep white matter (*arrow*). Note: In contrast to MS, lesions in ADEM have often poorly defined margins. ADEM tends to spare periventricular white matter, but 30–60% of the patients may have some involvement of this area

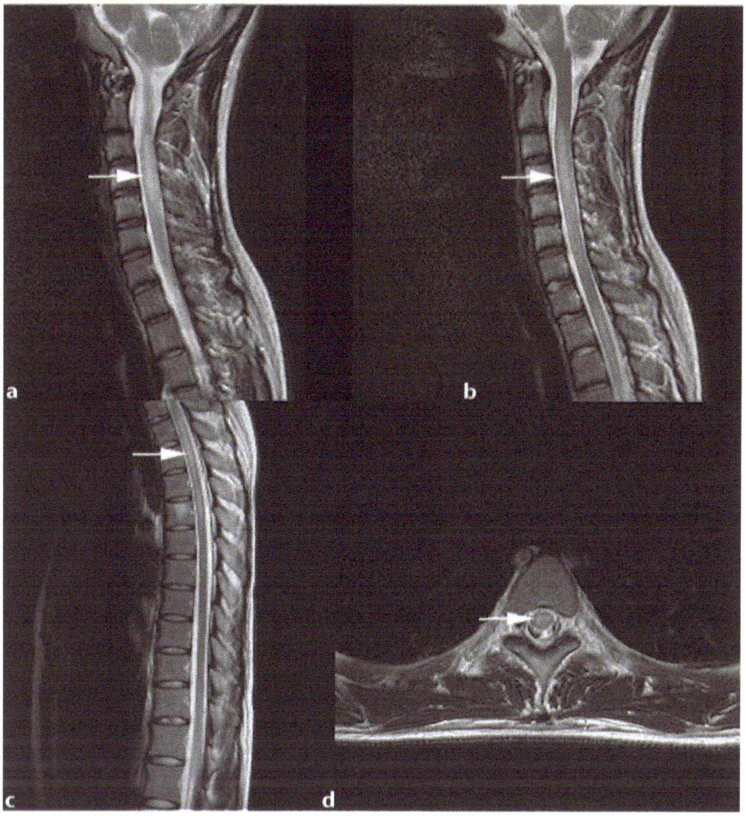

Fig. 9.16 Sagittal PD- (**a**,**b**), T1-weighted with contrast (**c**,**d**) images of cervical (**a**,**b**) and thoracic (**c**) spinal cord of a patient with ADEM demonstrate spinal cord involvement (*arrows*). Note: In most patients spinal lesions occur together with cerebral lesions. Spinal lesions are not specific and are indistinguishable from MS lesions; however, spinal lesions in ADEM tend to extend over more segments of the cord

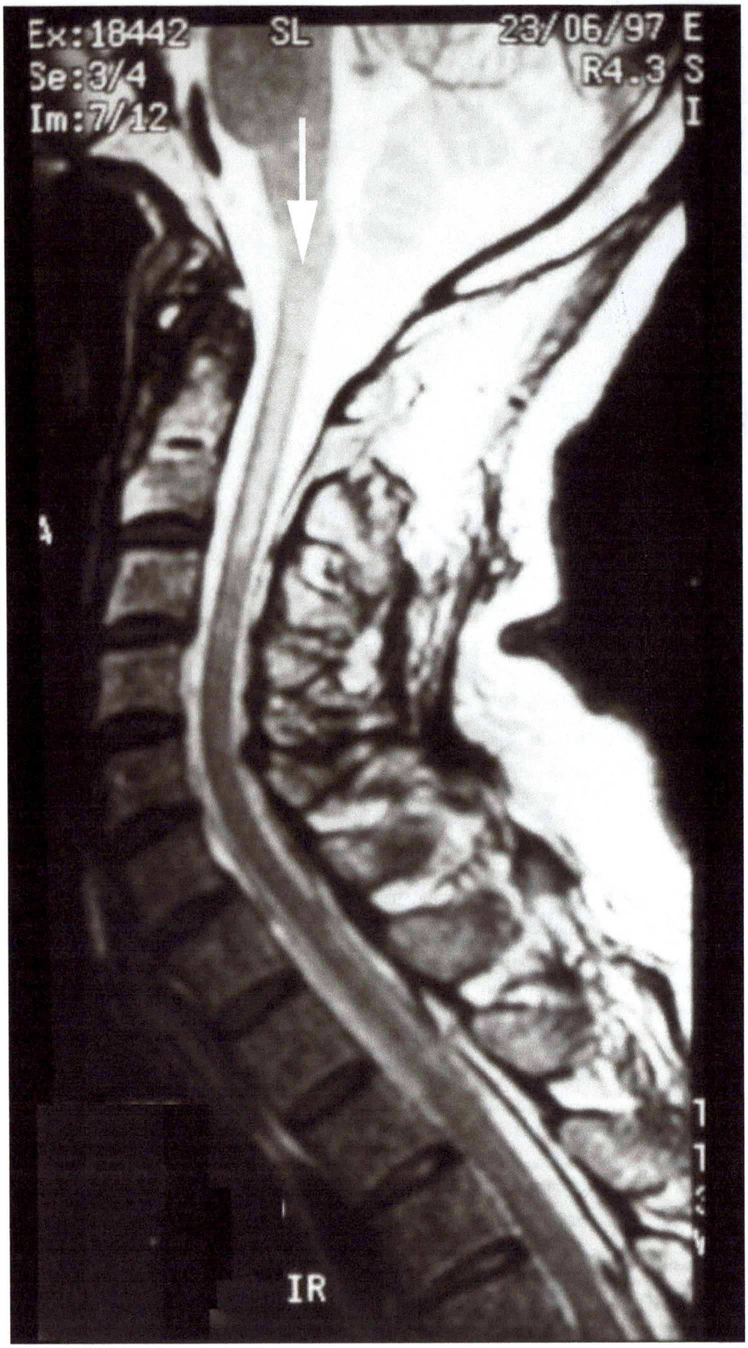

Fig. 9.17 Sagittal T2-weighted image of a patient with Devic's disease demonstrate a hyperintense lesion in the cervical part of the spinal cord. Note: Spinal lesions in Devic's disease tend to be more extensive, involving more than three vertebral segments

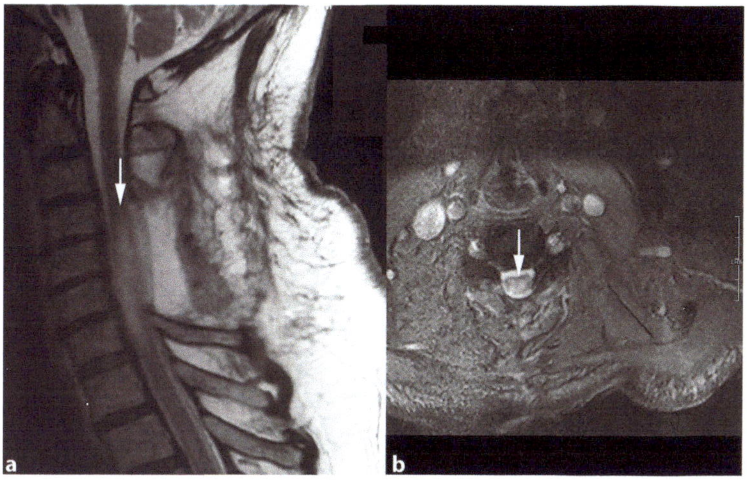

Fig. 9.18 Sagittal T2-weighted (**a**) and axial (**b**) images of a patient with Devic's disease demonstrate a hyperintense lesion in the cervical part of the spinal cord, which exceeds two vertebral segments of the cord. Note: Diagnosis of Devic's disease needs clinical experience of myelitis, optic neuritis and two of the following features: (1) normal or nonspecific brain MRI, (2) spinal lesion extending more than three vertebral segments, and (3) presence of neuromyelitis optica IgG

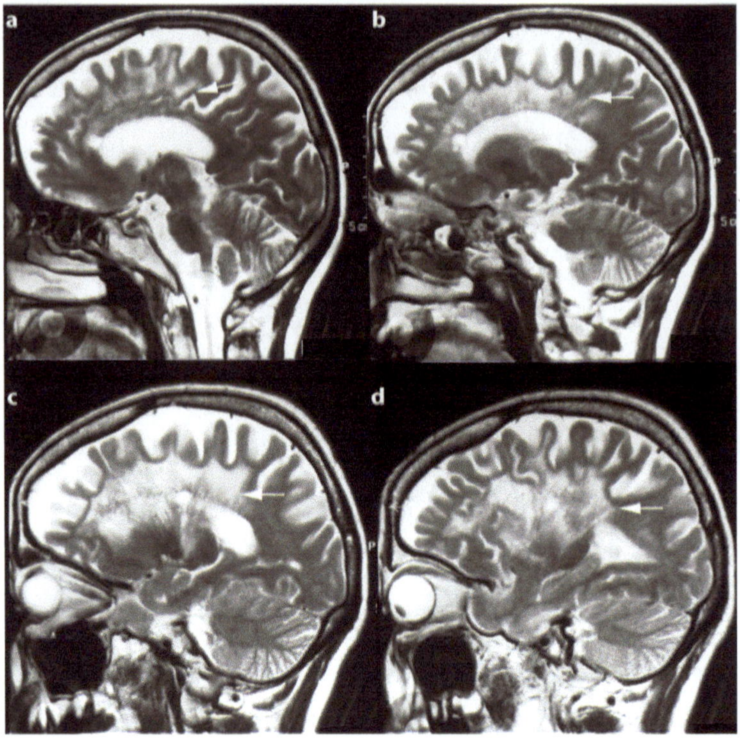

Fig. 9.19 Sagittal selected images of a patient with Schilder's disease demonstrate severe involvement of white matter (*arrows*). Note: Schilder's disease is a rare demyelinating disorder with an earlier age of onset that often results in severe neurological deficits. Brain MRI may reveal bilateral large hemispheric lesions with involvement of the corpus callosum and peripheral enhancement

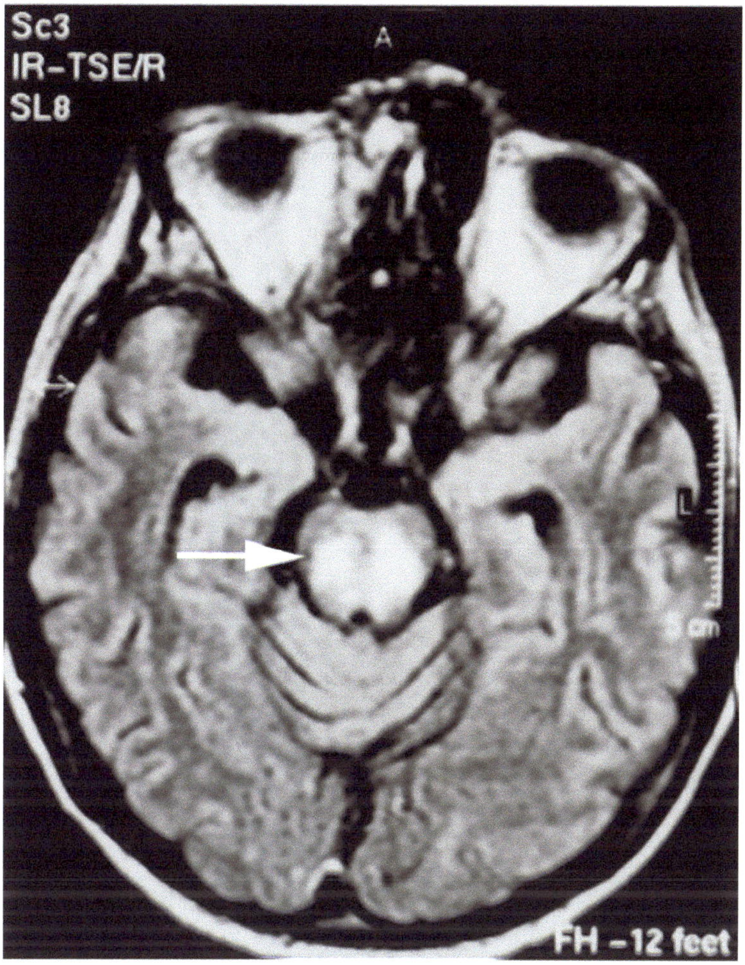

Fig. 9.20 Axial FLAIR image of a patient with central pontine myelinolysis, demonstrating a central area of signal changes within the pons without corresponding mass effect (*arrow*)

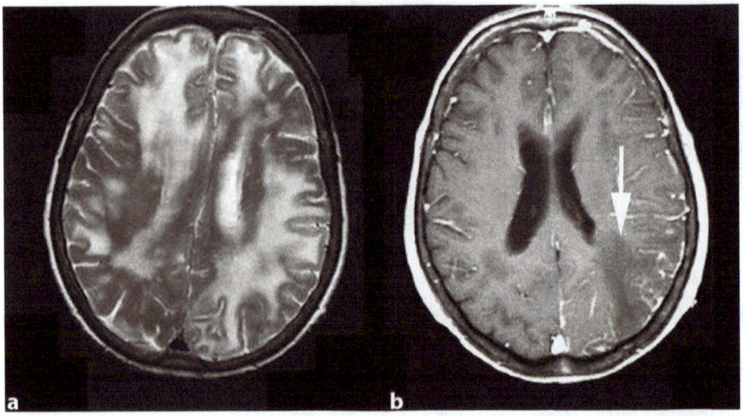

Fig. 9.21 Axial T2-weighted (**a**) and T1-weighted with contrast (**b**) images of a patient with PML demonstrate severe bilateral cerebral involvement. The lesions have no mass effect, do not enhance after contrast injection, and are not symmetrical

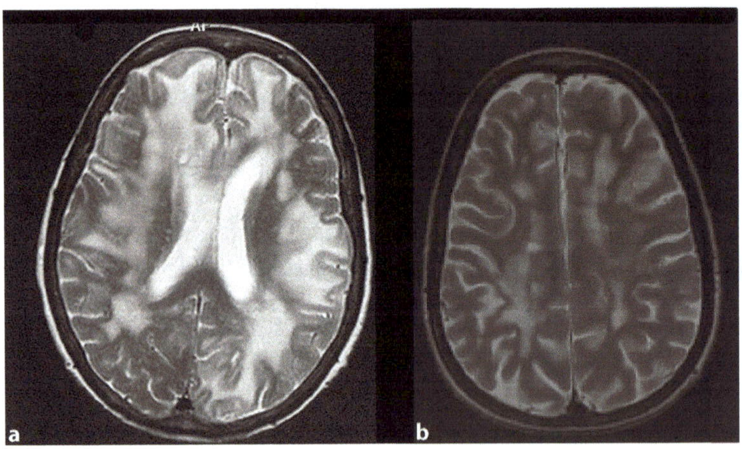

Fig. 9.22 Axial T2-weighted image of a patient with PML (**a**) and PD image of a patient with MS. The following features help in differentiation: (1) relative sparing of periventricular area in PML, (2) severe destruction of U-fibers, and (3) poorly defined borders of the lesions in PML

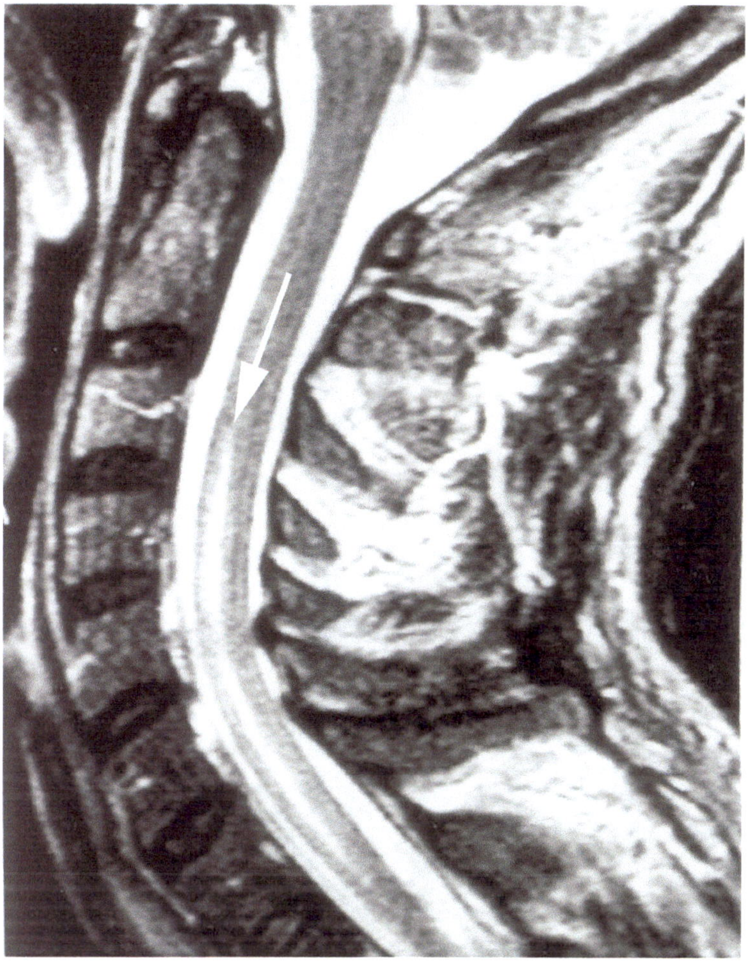

Fig. 9.23 Sagittal T2-weighted image of a patient with Lyme disease demonstrate a long hyperintense lesion involving cervical and thoracic parts of the spinal cord. Note the antromedial involvement of the cord

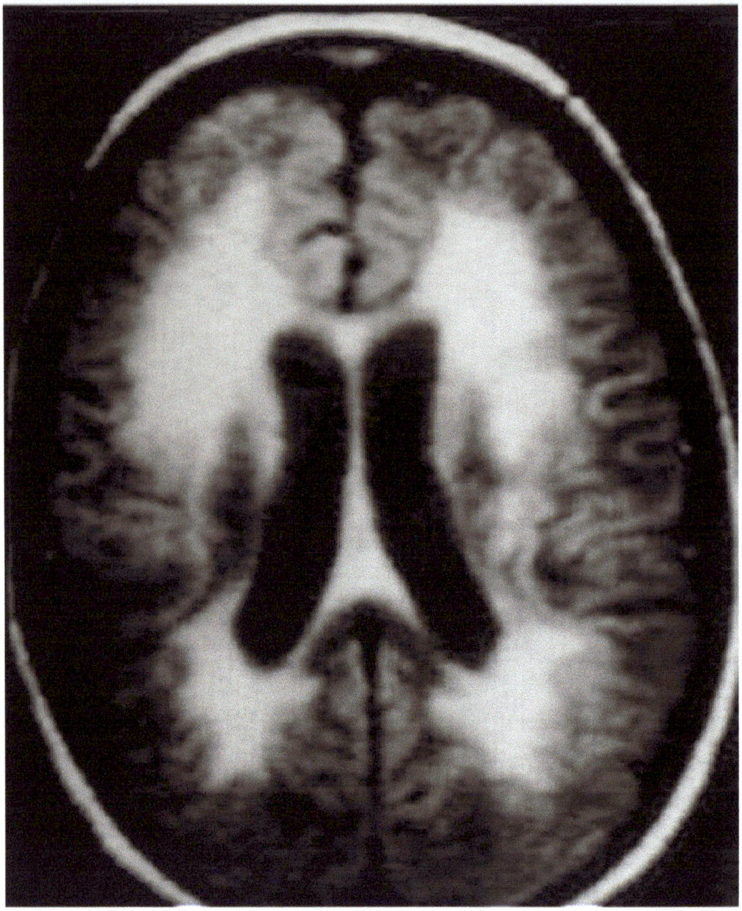

Fig. 9.24 Axial FLAIR image of a patient with adrenoleukodystrophy demonstrates bilateral symmetrical involvement of white matter. Note: Inherited metabolic diseases that involve the brain are usually bilateral and symmetrical. Adrenoleukodystrophy shows contrast enhancement

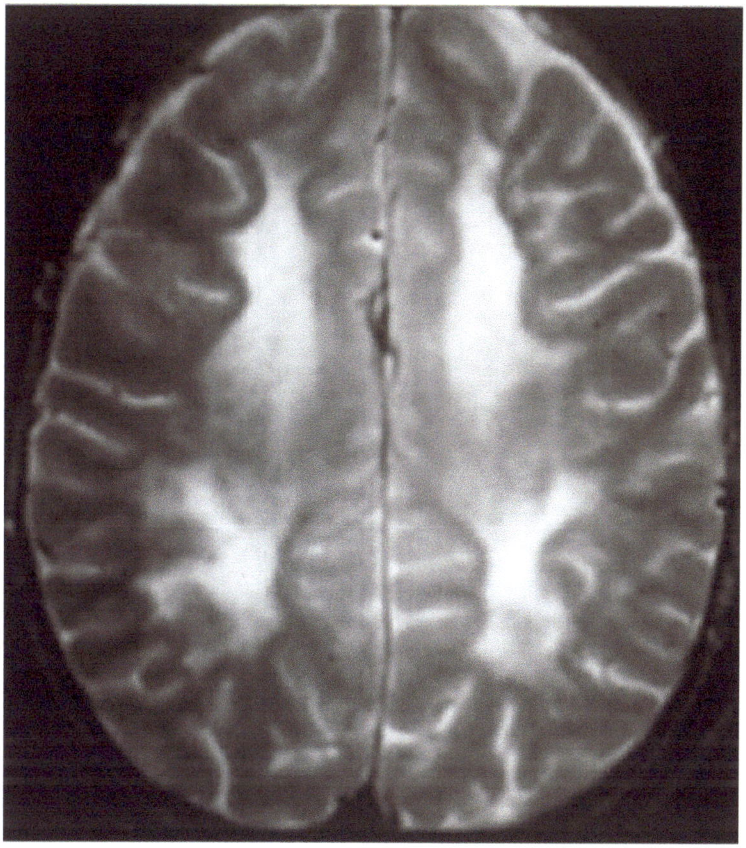

Fig. 9.25 Axial T2-weighted image of a patient with metachromatic leukodystrophy demonstrates bilateral symmetrical involvement of the white matter. Note: Widespread, symmetrical, confluent lesions, sparing U-fibers help in differentiating from MS. The pattern of involvement is periventricular, bilateral and symmetrical (butterfly pattern). The lesions do not enhance after Gd injection

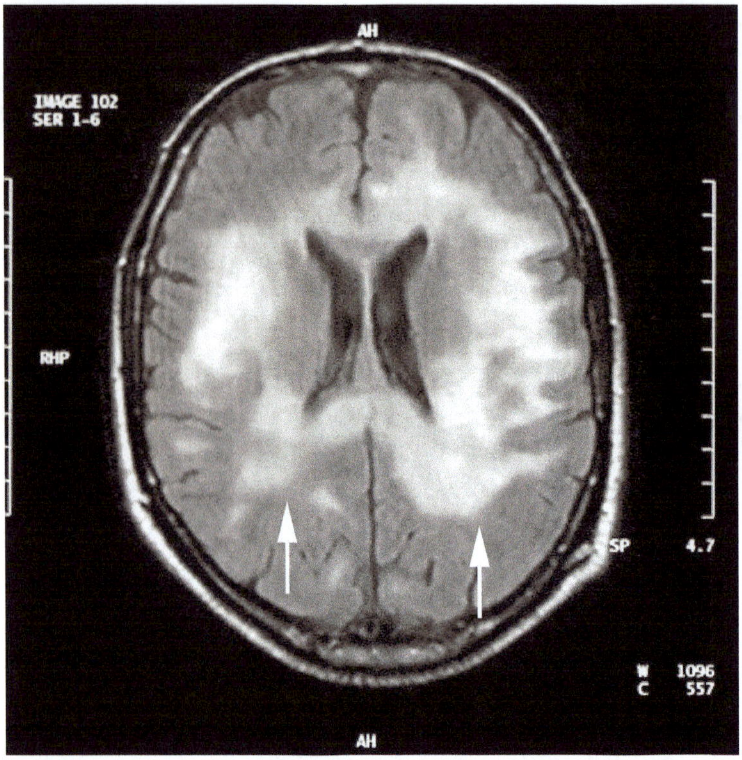

Fig. 9.26 Axial FLAIR image of a patient with post radiation encephalopathy demonstrates severe diffuse leukoencephalopathy after radiation. Note: White matter damage may occur after cranial or spinal irradiation. MRI reveals severe white matter damage that is usually bilateral

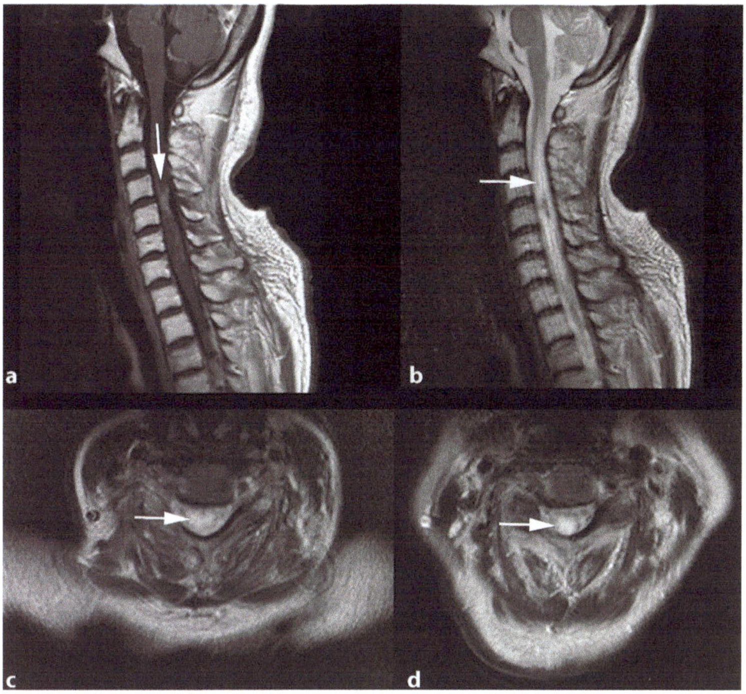

Fig 9.27 Sagittal T1-weighted with contrast (**a**) and T2-weighted (**b**) images of a patient with breast cancer and bone metastasis who had radiation. The patient developed radiation myelopathy 1 year after radiotherapy. Note: Focal cord swelling with Gd enhancement has been described in post radiation myelopathy. This diagnosis should be considered in patients with history of radiotherapy

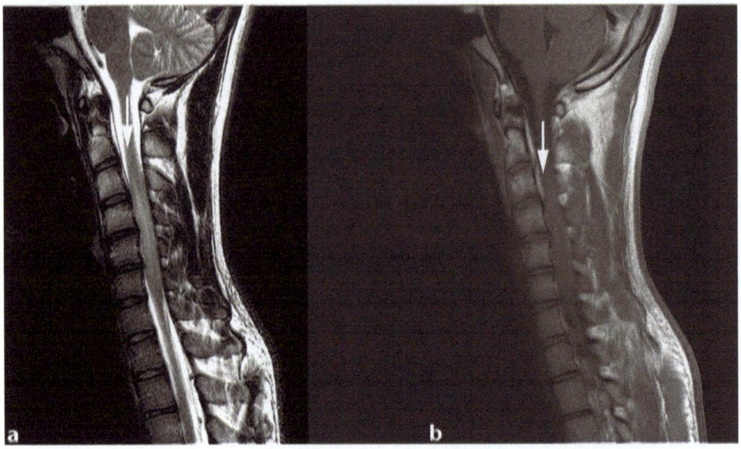

Fig. 9.28 Sagittal T2-weighted (**a**) and T1-weigthed with contrast (**b**) images of a patient with astrocytoma of the spinal cord. The lesion is hyperintense on the T2-weighted image and has not enhanced after contrast injection. Note: Tumors are usually associated with swelling of the cord, whereas MS causes atrophy of the spinal cord. This lesion has extended over more than two vertebral segments, which is not typical for MS

References

1. Akman-Demir G, Serdaroglu P, Tasci B (1999) Clinical patterns of neurological involvement in Behçet's disease: evaluation of 200 patients. The Neuro-Behçet Study Group. Brain 122:2171–2182
2. Barkhof F, Scheltens P (2002) Imaging of white matter lesions. Cerebrovasc Dis 13(Suppl 2):21–30
3. Berger JR, Houff S (2006) Progressive multifocal leukoencephalopathy: lessons from AIDS and natalizumab. Neurol Res 28:299–305
4. Borhani Haghighi A, Pourmand R, Nikseresht AR (2005) Neuro-Behçet disease. Neurologist 11:80–89
5. Dale RC, Branson JA (2005) Acute disseminated encephalomyelitis or multiple sclerosis: can the initial presentation help in establishing a correct diagnosis? Arch Dis Child 90:636–639
6. Douen AG, Pringle CE, Guberman A (1997) Human T-cell lymphotropic virus type 1 myositis, peripheral neuropathy, and cerebral white matter lesions in the absence of spastic paraparesis. Arch Neurol 54:896–900
7. Drayer BP (1988) Imaging of the aging brain. Part I. Normal findings. Radiology 166:785–796
8. Filippi M, Rocca MA (2004) MR imaging of Devic's neuromyelitis optica. Neurol Sci 25(Suppl 4):S371–S373
9. Gasperini C (2001) Differential diagnosis in multiple sclerosis. Neurol Sci 22(Suppl 2):S93–S97
10. Gullapalli D, Phillips LH II (2002) Neurologic manifestations of sarcoidosis. Neurol Clin 20:59–83

11. Hynson JL, Kornberg AJ, Coleman LT et al (2001) Clinical and neuroradiologic features of acute disseminated encephalomyelitis in children. Neurology 56:1308–1312
12. Ijichi S, Osame M (1995) Human T lymphotropic virus type I (HTLV-I)-associated myelopathy/tropical spastic paraparesis (HAM/TSP): recent perspectives. Intern Med 34:713–721
13. Isella V, Marzorati L, Curto N et al (2005) Primary progressive multifocal leukoencephalopathy: report of a case. Funct Neurol 20:139–42
14. Kapeller P, Schmidt R, Fazekas F (2004) Qualitative MRI: evidence of usual aging in the brain. Top Magn Reson Imaging 15:343–3471
15. Koralnik IJ (2004) New insights into progressive multifocal leukoencephalopathy. Curr Opin Neurol 17:365–370
16. Lampl C, Yazdi K (2002) Central pontine myelinolysis. Eur Neurol 47:3–10
17. Lexa FJ, Grossman RI (1994) MR of sarcoidosis in the head and spine: spectrum of manifestations and radiographic response to steroid therapy. AJNR Am J Neuroradiol 15:973–982
18. Loeb C (2000) Binswanger›s disease is not a single entity. Neurol Sci 21:343–348
19. Major EO, Amemiya K, Tornatore CS et al (1992) Pathogenesis and molecular biology of progressive multifocal leukoencephalopathy, the JC virus-induced demyelinating disease of the human brain. Clin Microbiol Rev 5:49–73
20. Murthy SN, Faden HS, Cohen ME (2002) Acute disseminated encephalomyelitis in children. Pediatrics 110(2 Pt 1):e21
21. Nachman SA, Pontrelli L (2003) Central nervous system Lyme disease. Semin Pediatr Infect Dis 14:123–130
22. Norenberg MD, Leslie KO, Robertson AS (1982) Association between rise in serum sodium and central pontine myelinolysis. Ann Neurol 11:128–135
23. Rosen L, Phillips S, Enzmann D (1990) Magnetic resonance imaging in MELAS syndrome. Neuroradiology 32:168–171
24. Sharma (1997) Neurosarcoidosis a personal perspective based on the study of 37 patients. Chest 112:220–228
25. Spencer TS, Campellone JV, Maldonado I et al (2005) Clinical and magnetic resonance imaging manifestations of neurosarcoidosis. Semin Arthritis Rheum 34:649–661
26. Tenembaum S, Chamoles N, Fejerman N (2002) Acute disseminated encephalomyelitis: a long-term follow-up study of 84 pediatric patients. Neurology 59:1224–1231
27. Thurnher MM, Thurnher SA, Muhlbauer B et al (1997) Progressive multifocal leukoencephalopathy in AIDS: initial and follow-up CT and MRI. Neuroradiology 39:611–618
28. Trojano M, Paolicelli D (2001) The differential diagnosis of multiple sclerosis: classification and clinical features of relapsing and progressive neurological syndromes. Neurol Sci 22(Suppl 2):S98–S102
29. Vanzieleghem B, Lemmerling M, Carton D et al (1998) Lyme disease in a child presenting with bilateral facial nerve palsy: MRI findings and review of the literature. Neuroradiology 40:739–742
30. Vikelis M, Xifaras M, Mitsikostas DD (2006) CADASIL: a short review of the literature and a description of the first family from Greece. Funct Neurol 21:77–82
31. Wingerchuk DM (2007) Diagnosis and treatment of neuromyelitis optica. Neurologist 13:2–11
32. Yousry TA, Major EO, Ryschkewitsch C et al (2006) Evaluation of patients treated with natalizumab for progressive multifocal leukoencephalopathy. N Engl J Med 354:924–933

Subject Index

Please note: Anatomical structures are referred to as locations of MS lesions.

MIX
Papier aus verantwortungsvollen Quellen
Paper from responsible sources
FSC® C105338

If you have any concerns about our products,
you can contact us on
ProductSafety@springernature.com

In case Publisher is established outside the EU,
the EU authorized representative is:
Springer Nature Customer Service Center GmbH
Europaplatz 3, 69115 Heidelberg, Germany

Printed by Libri Plureos GmbH
in Hamburg, Germany